21st CENTURY INVENTIONS

MEDICAL and ADVANCED INVENTIONS

WORLD BOOK

www.worldbook.com

Co-published by agreement between Shi Tu Hui and World Book, Inc.

Shi Tu Hui
Room 1807, Block 1,
#3 West Dawang Road
Chaoyang District, Beijing 100025
P.R. China

World Book, Inc.
180 North LaSalle Street
Suite 900
Chicago, Illinois 60601
USA

© 2025. All rights reserved. This volume may not be reproduced in whole or in part in any form without prior written permission from the publisher.

WORLD BOOK and the GLOBE DEVICE are registered trademarks or trademarks of World Book, Inc.

Library of Congress Control Number: 2024943009

21st Century Inventions
ISBN: 978-0-7166-5360-8 (set, hard cover)

Medical and Advanced Inventions
ISBN: 978-0-7166-5361-5 (hard cover)
ISBN: 978-0-7166-5367-7 (e-book)
ISBN: 978-0-7166-5364-6 (soft cover)

WORLD BOOK STAFF

Editorial

Vice President
Tom Evans

Senior Manager, New Content
Jeff De La Rosa

Manager, New Product Development
Nicholas Kilzer

Content Creator
Elizabeth Huyck

Writers
William D. Adams
Lauren Kelliher
Fred Maxon
Jenna Neely

Proofreader
Nathalie Strassheim

Indexer
Nathaniel Lindstrom

Graphics and Design

Senior Visual Communications Designer
Melanie Bender

Digital Asset Specialist
Rosalia Bledsoe

Acknowledgments
Designer: Starletta Polster
Writer: Alex Woolf

CONTENTS

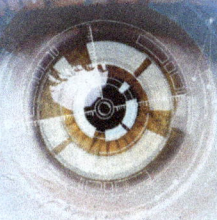

3D printed organs 4
Aerogels 6
Artificial intelligence 8
Artificial liver 12
Bionics 14
Brain-computer interface 16
Cloned monkeys 18
Cloud computing 20
CRISPR 22
CubeSats 26
Event Horizon Telescope 28
Foods from genetically modified animals 30
Holograms 32
Home genetic testing 34
Human genome 38
Infrared thermometer 40
James Webb Space Telescope 42
Lab-grown meat 46
Large Hadron Collider 48
Laser Interferometer Gravitational-Wave Observatory (LIGO) ... 50
Metamaterials 52
mRNA vaccines 54
Personal insulin pump 56
Prosthetics 58
Quantum computing 62
Retinal implants 64
Reusable rockets 66
Satellite internet 68
Solid-state lidar 70
Space crops 72
Telehealth 74
Wireless capsule endoscopy 76
Index 78
Acknowledgments 80

3D printed organs:
Organs made to order

Wouldn't it be great if a doctor could order you a new lung or liver—just like writing a prescription? It may soon be possible through 3D printing. Three-dimensional (3D) printing can create three-dimensional (3D) objects from computer models.

If an organ is damaged through injury, disease, or old age, it can be replaced in an organ transplant operation. The replacement organ must come from a donor. But there are not enough donor organs to go around. In addition, the patient's body sometimes rejects the donor organ. Made-to-order organs could help solve both these problems.

Scientists are developing several methods for 3D printing organs and body tissues. In one method, doctors will take small samples of organ tissues from the patient's body. Then they will place each type of tissue in a device called a bioreactor. Inside the bioreactors, each tissue type will divide and grow. Then, the doctors will mix each type with a special glue and load the mixture into a medical 3D printer. The printer will build the organ up by depositing tissue one layer at a time.

Finally, doctors will operate to replace the damaged organ with the newly printed one. After the surgery, the glue holding the cells together will slowly *dissolve* (melt away). As it does, the cells will grow connections to their neighbors.

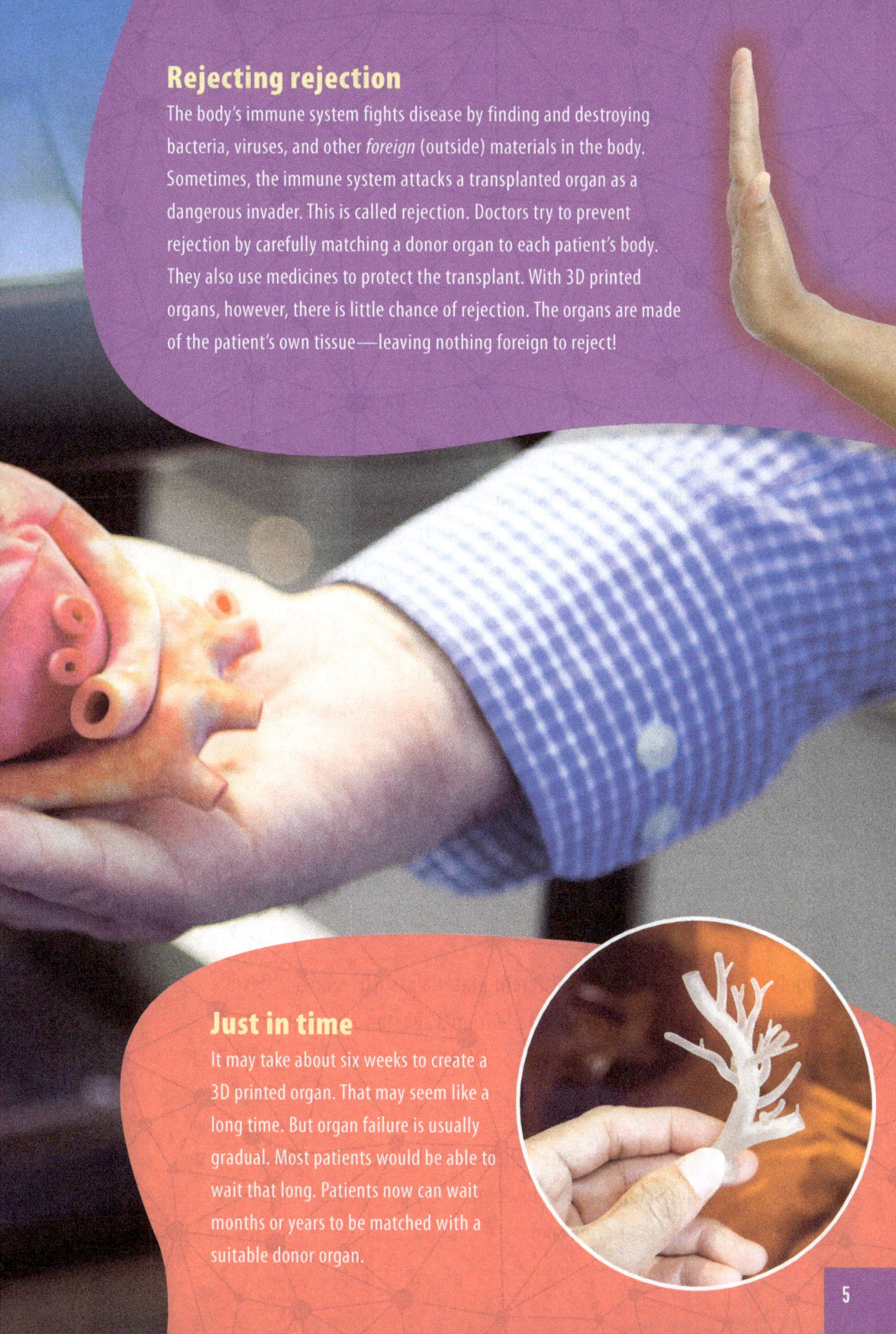

Rejecting rejection

The body's immune system fights disease by finding and destroying bacteria, viruses, and other *foreign* (outside) materials in the body. Sometimes, the immune system attacks a transplanted organ as a dangerous invader. This is called rejection. Doctors try to prevent rejection by carefully matching a donor organ to each patient's body. They also use medicines to protect the transplant. With 3D printed organs, however, there is little chance of rejection. The organs are made of the patient's own tissue—leaving nothing foreign to reject!

Just in time

It may take about six weeks to create a 3D printed organ. That may seem like a long time. But organ failure is usually gradual. Most patients would be able to wait that long. Patients now can wait months or years to be matched with a suitable donor organ.

AEROGELS:
Solid clouds

Imagine you need to create a spacesuit. The material you choose must protect an astronaut from the extreme heat and cold of space. It must also be light and thin so the astronaut can easily move around. How about an aerogel?

An aerogel is like a sponge with millions of tiny holes called pores. Each pore is far smaller than the width of a human hair. Aerogels have so many pores that about 95 to 99 percent of their volume is air. This makes them some of the lightest materials ever made. It's no wonder they are sometimes called "frozen smoke" or "solid clouds."

Under a microscope, an aerogel looks like a maze of pathways around the pores. This makes it hard for air to move through the material, so aerogels are good insulators (materials that block the flow of heat).

To make an aerogel, you first make a gel—a mixture of a liquid and a solid. The solid part forms a lattice that holds the liquid in place. When the gel is subjected to high temperature and pressure, the liquid turns to gas and escapes. This leaves a solid aerogel behind.

Aerogels can be made into many different materials, such as bricks, flexible sheets, or thin coatings. An aerogel made from a substance that attracts certain molecules can be used as an air or water filter. An aerogel called silica gel can remove water from the air.

Some aerogels are *translucent*—they allow some light to pass through. These aerogels are ideal for insulating windows and solar panels. They can even cover bottles, keeping your drink cool.

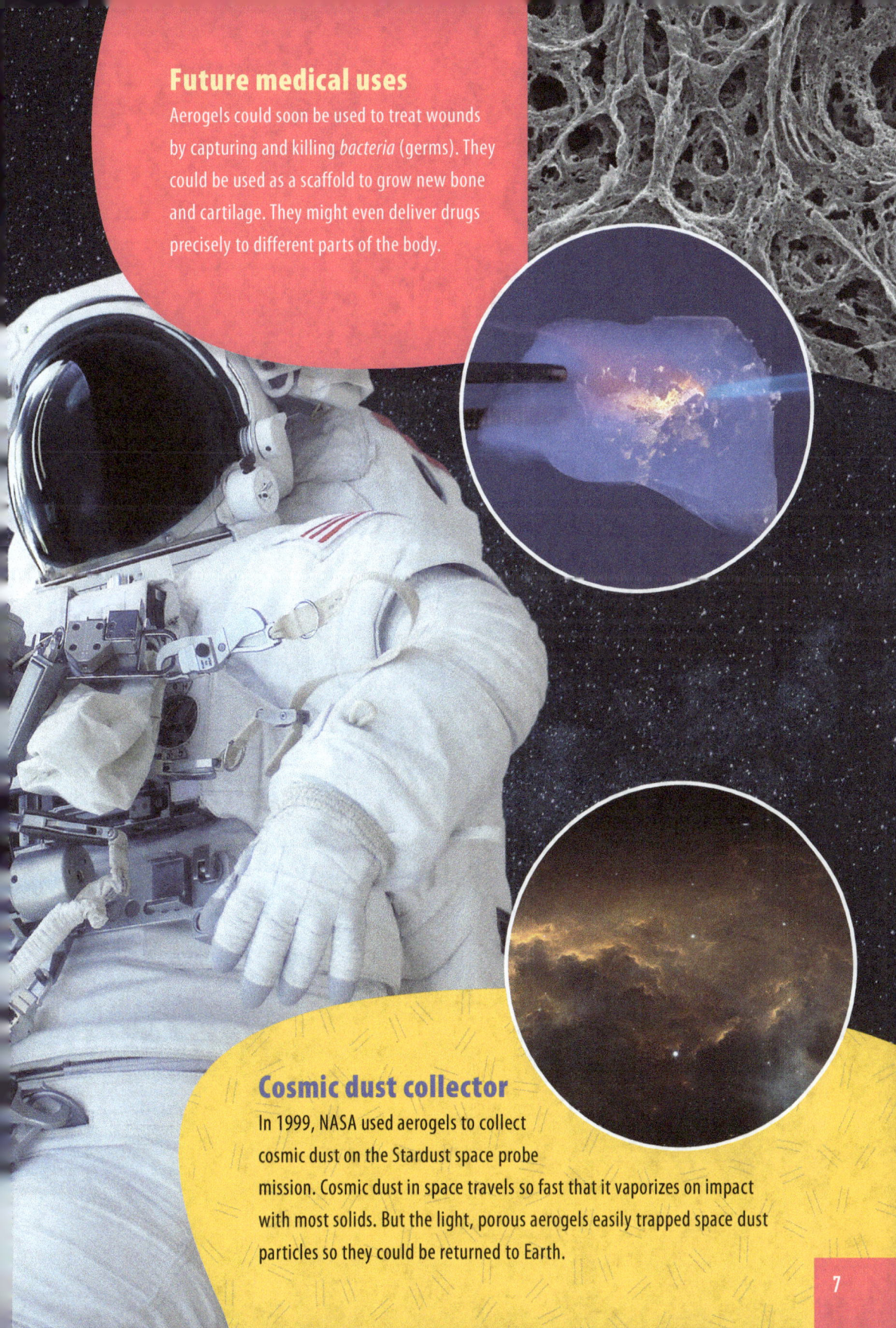

Future medical uses

Aerogels could soon be used to treat wounds by capturing and killing *bacteria* (germs). They could be used as a scaffold to grow new bone and cartilage. They might even deliver drugs precisely to different parts of the body.

Cosmic dust collector

In 1999, NASA used aerogels to collect cosmic dust on the Stardust space probe mission. Cosmic dust in space travels so fast that it vaporizes on impact with most solids. But the light, porous aerogels easily trapped space dust particles so they could be returned to Earth.

Artificial Intelligence:
Machines that think

Might it be possible one day to build a machine with the intelligence and emotional awareness of a human? Such a machine could help you with everyday tasks, offer advice, or simply be a friend. This may be the ultimate goal of what we call *artificial intelligence* (AI). We're not there yet, but we're making good progress. Today, AI is helping us in many different ways, and it's getting better all the time.

AI is a field of science concerned with building machines that can think like humans. This means being able to learn, reason, identify patterns, perceive objects, and understand language.

The simplest form of AI is known as reactive AI. This uses an *algorithm* (a sequence of instructions) to carry out tasks. It is unable to learn new actions and will always react predictably. An email spam filter is an example of a reactive AI.

A more advanced form of AI is called machine learning. This uses data to make connections, discover patterns, and make predictions. It can learn and improve on its own, with no need for human input. A machine-learning algorithm could, for example, learn what a cat looks like by examining lots of pictures of cats.

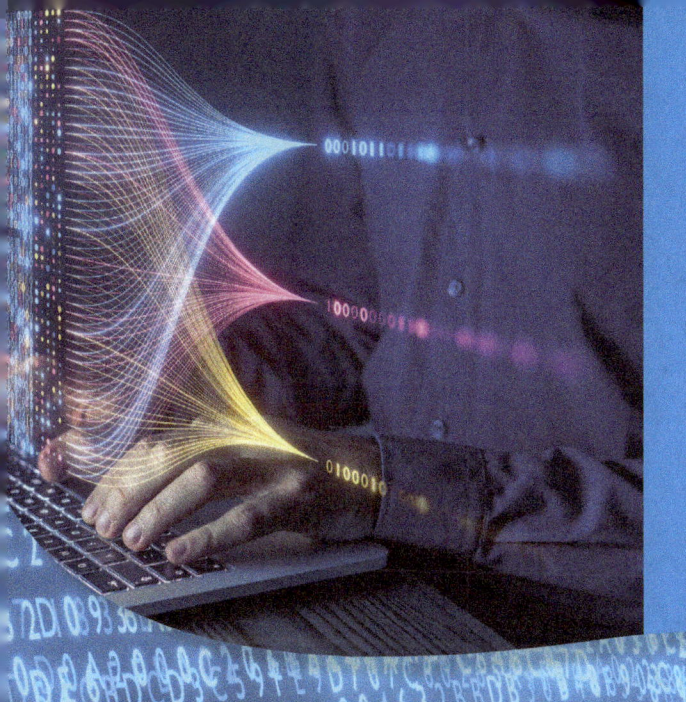

Strong and weak AI

AI is often divided into two categories: weak and strong. Weak AI does a single task very well. This is the kind of AI mostly in use today. Examples include virtual assistants, music-streaming recommendations, and chess-playing computers. Strong AI would be AI with a humanlike intelligence that could apply itself to any task. Such an AI may be possible in theory, but no one has built one yet.

From Turing to ChatGPT

In 1950, British computer scientist Alan Turing predicted that computers would one day become intelligent, and he proposed a test that could tell humans and computers apart. In 1956, American computer scientist John McCarthy coined the term *artificial intelligence*. The first artificial neural networks were developed in the 1980's. In 1997, a computer called Deep Blue defeated the world chess champion Garry Kasparov in a chess match. By the 2020's, such AI large language models as ChatGPT could generate written text that closely mimics humans.

The human brain contains millions of interconnected neurons that work together to process information. Deep-learning algorithms do the same with an artificial neural network.

When a deep-learning AI receives information (input), hundreds of hidden layers process the data. They also adapt as new data is added. If the algorithm is attempting to identify cats, for example, and it finds whiskers in an image, it will assign that image a higher "cat" value because it has encountered whiskers in previous cat pictures. These programs often make mistakes, but the more images the network analyzes, the more accurate it becomes.

This is how it "learns."

Deep learning is very good at finding patterns in large amounts of raw data. It is useful for detecting financial fraud, identifying a tumor in a medical scan, or recommending a movie based on a person's viewing history.

Every time you use social media, a navigation app, or a fitness tracker, you are using AI. Virtual assistants and chatbots use a form of AI called *natural language processing* to understand and respond to ordinary speech. Today, artists, musicians, and writers use AI models to generate ideas and help them with projects.

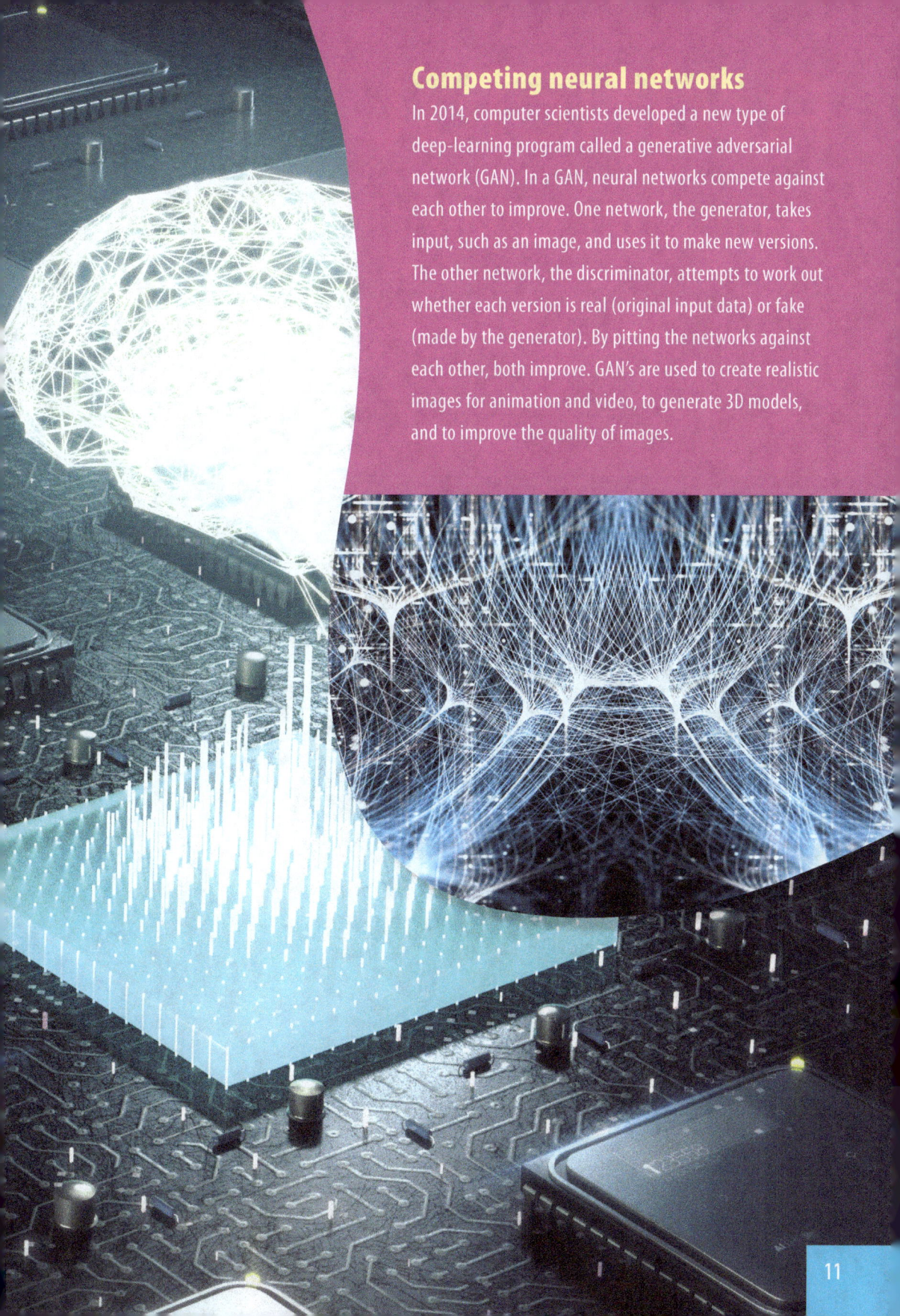

Competing neural networks

In 2014, computer scientists developed a new type of deep-learning program called a generative adversarial network (GAN). In a GAN, neural networks compete against each other to improve. One network, the generator, takes input, such as an image, and uses it to make new versions. The other network, the discriminator, attempts to work out whether each version is real (original input data) or fake (made by the generator). By pitting the networks against each other, both improve. GAN's are used to create realistic images for animation and video, to generate 3D models, and to improve the quality of images.

Artificial liver:
A substitute organ

The liver is one of the most complex organs in the human body. It helps the body turn food into energy, makes bile to break down fats, and filters poisons and waste from the blood. The liver is the only human organ that can regenerate itself. Yet nearly 2 million people around the world die from liver failure each year.

Scientists have searched tirelessly for ways to help. In 2001, the American oncologist Kenneth Matsumura invented a way to use liver cells (called hepatocytes) from rabbits to do the liver's job outside of the body. He called it the bio-artificial liver.

The bio-artificial liver has two chambers. A patient's blood flows in one chamber. The other holds rabbit hepatocytes. A semipermeable membrane between the chambers allows the rabbit cells to remove toxins and waste from the blood. But rabbit cells never touch human cells. This prevents infection or rejection, where the body fights off unknown cells.

The bio-artificial liver is not a long-term solution in its current state. It is designed to keep patients healthy while they wait for a liver transplant or while the liver heals. But researchers hope that this life-saving invention will lead to more innovation.

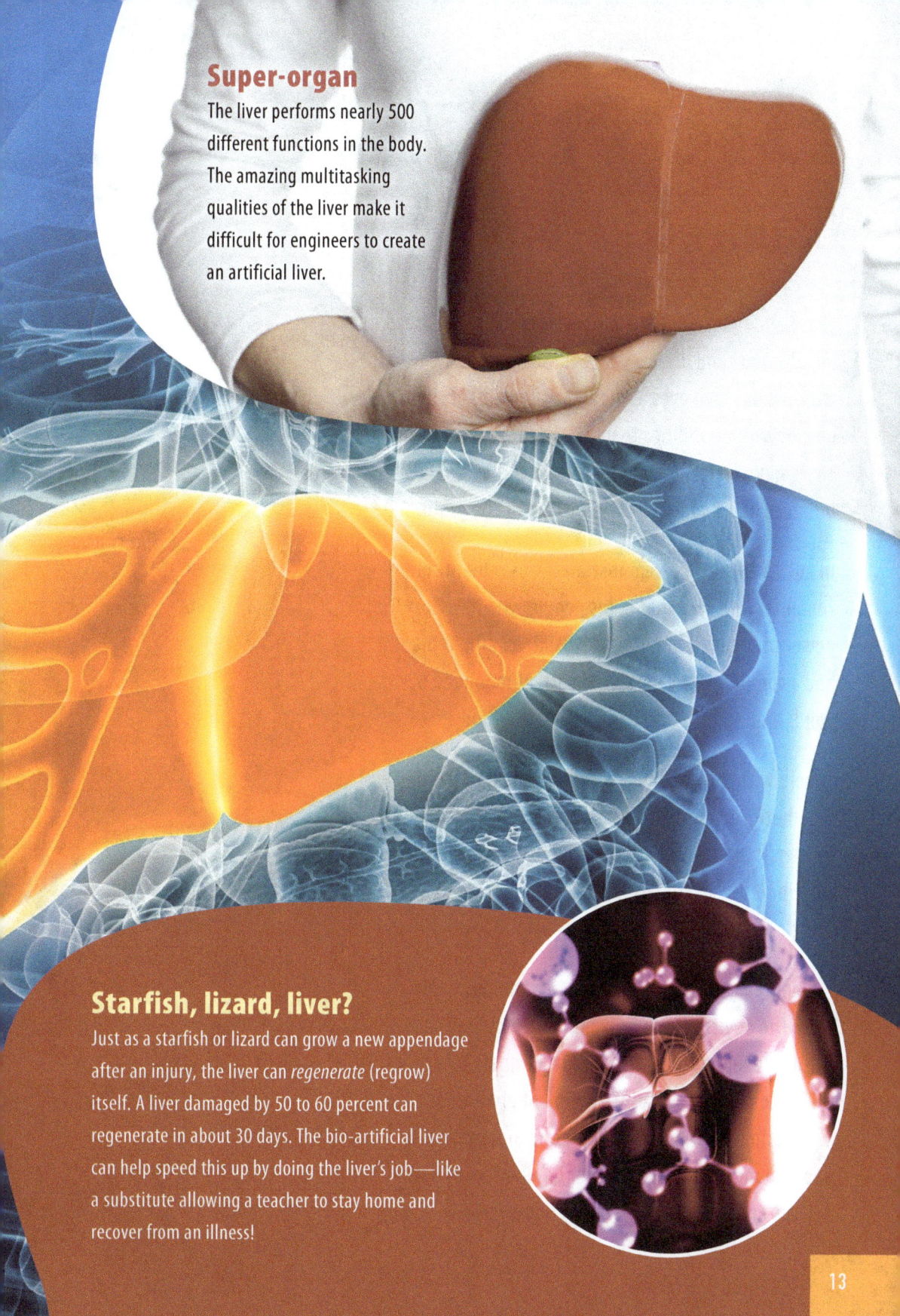

Super-organ
The liver performs nearly 500 different functions in the body. The amazing multitasking qualities of the liver make it difficult for engineers to create an artificial liver.

Starfish, lizard, liver?
Just as a starfish or lizard can grow a new appendage after an injury, the liver can *regenerate* (regrow) itself. A liver damaged by 50 to 60 percent can regenerate in about 30 days. The bio-artificial liver can help speed this up by doing the liver's job—like a substitute allowing a teacher to stay home and recover from an illness!

Bionics:
Brain-body connection

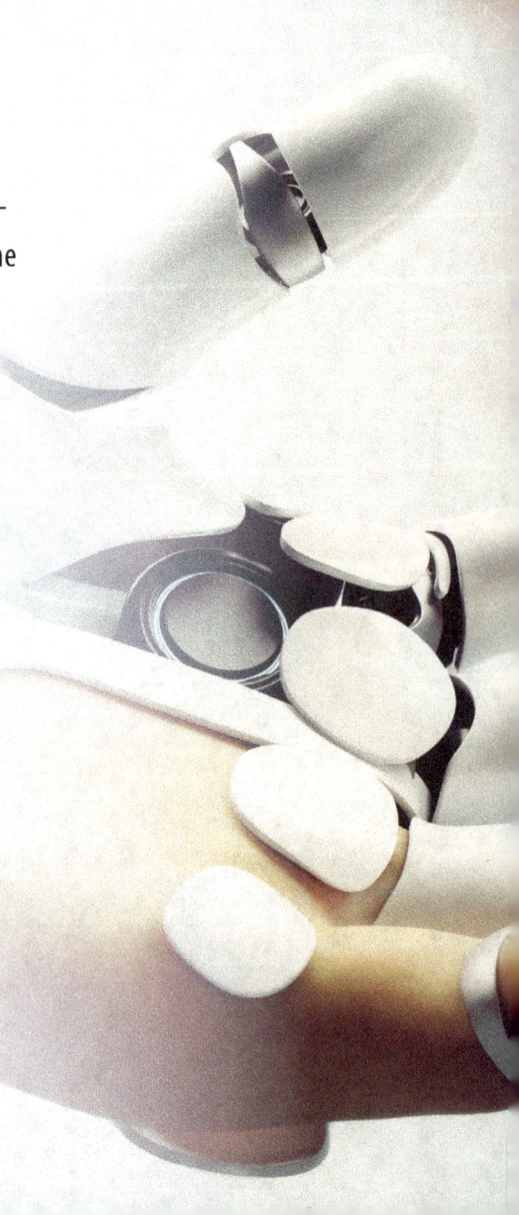

Sense and movement are important to everyday life. Some impairments and diseases take these abilities away. But today, super-cool eyes, ears, and body implants help people with disabilities to move, hear, see, and speak. These new devices are bionic—that is, they directly *interface* (work together) with nerves or the brain.

In 2023, researchers demonstrated a new bionic brain-computer interface that helps people who have lost the power of speech communicate. Using a brain implant and a computer, one paralyzed patient managed 62 words a minute, faster than previous methods.

People with missing limbs often replace them with prosthetic (artificial) body parts. A bionic limb goes farther. It interfaces with the body's neuromuscular system. It senses signals from the user's brain or muscles to bend, flex, or grasp.

A bionic ear called a cochlear implant helps people hear. The device is surgically implanted behind the ear. It converts sound into electrical signals, which generate nerve impulses. The implant enables people with serious hearing loss to hear and understand spoken language. Since the first implant in 1978, the sensors and processors have only improved.

Looking forward

The Orion Visual Cortical Prosthesis System was introduced in 2023 to help people with vision loss due to eye injury or disease to see again. Orion senses light and sends vision signals directly to the brain. The Argus II, below, is a bionic device that transmits visual information from a glasses-mounted camera to nerves in the user's retina, the light-sensitive tissue at the back of the eye.

Super suit

A bionic exoskeleton is like a wearable robot. Sensors in the suit detect small muscle movements or brain signals, and motors move the strong suit to match. This lets people with little or no muscle control walk and lift things. Exoskeletons can also help those recovering from strokes and spinal injuries.

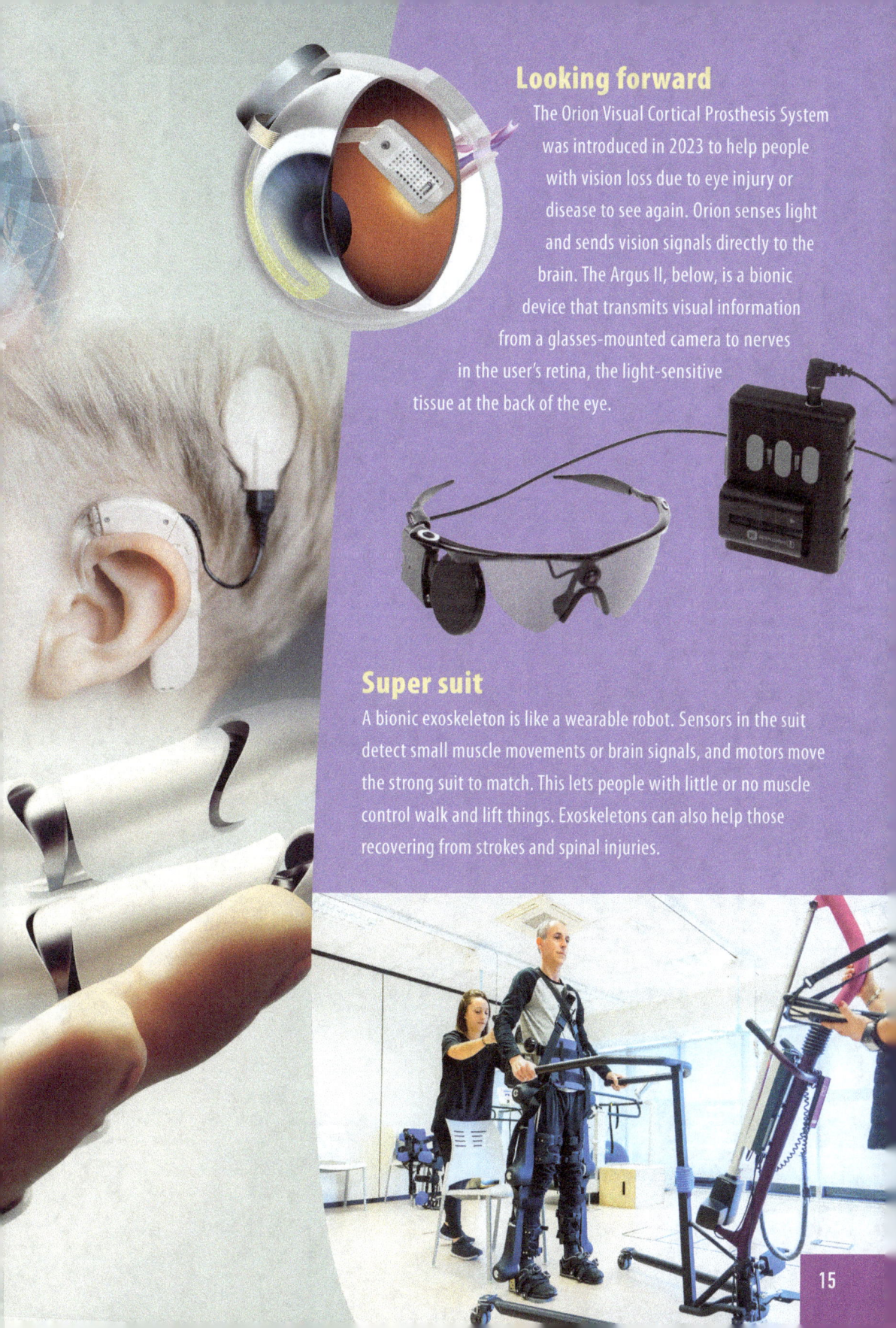

BRAIN-COMPUTER INTERFACE:

Controlling a machine with your thoughts

A thought flashes through a disabled person's head: *I want that apple*. Suddenly, their robotic *prosthetic* (replacement) arm is reaching for it. The idea of controlling a machine using only our thoughts sounds like science fiction. However, the technology is real, and is called brain-computer interface (BCI).

When you decide to throw a ball, your brain produces a certain pattern of electrical signals. Normally, nerves carry these impulses to your limbs. A BCI device can interpret these signals and pass instructions to a robotic limb instead. The interface detects brain signals using a cap fitted with sensors or a brain implant.

BCI technology can help people with prosthetic limbs to move and manipulate objects. People who have lost the ability to speak can use a BCI device to

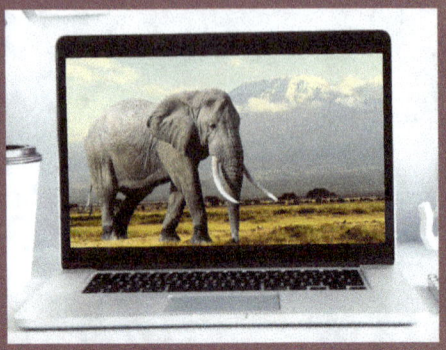

Mind pictures

A company called NextMind has been working on a device to turn our visual imagination into digital signals. So, for example, if you picture an elephant in your mind, the image of that elephant will appear on a computer screen.

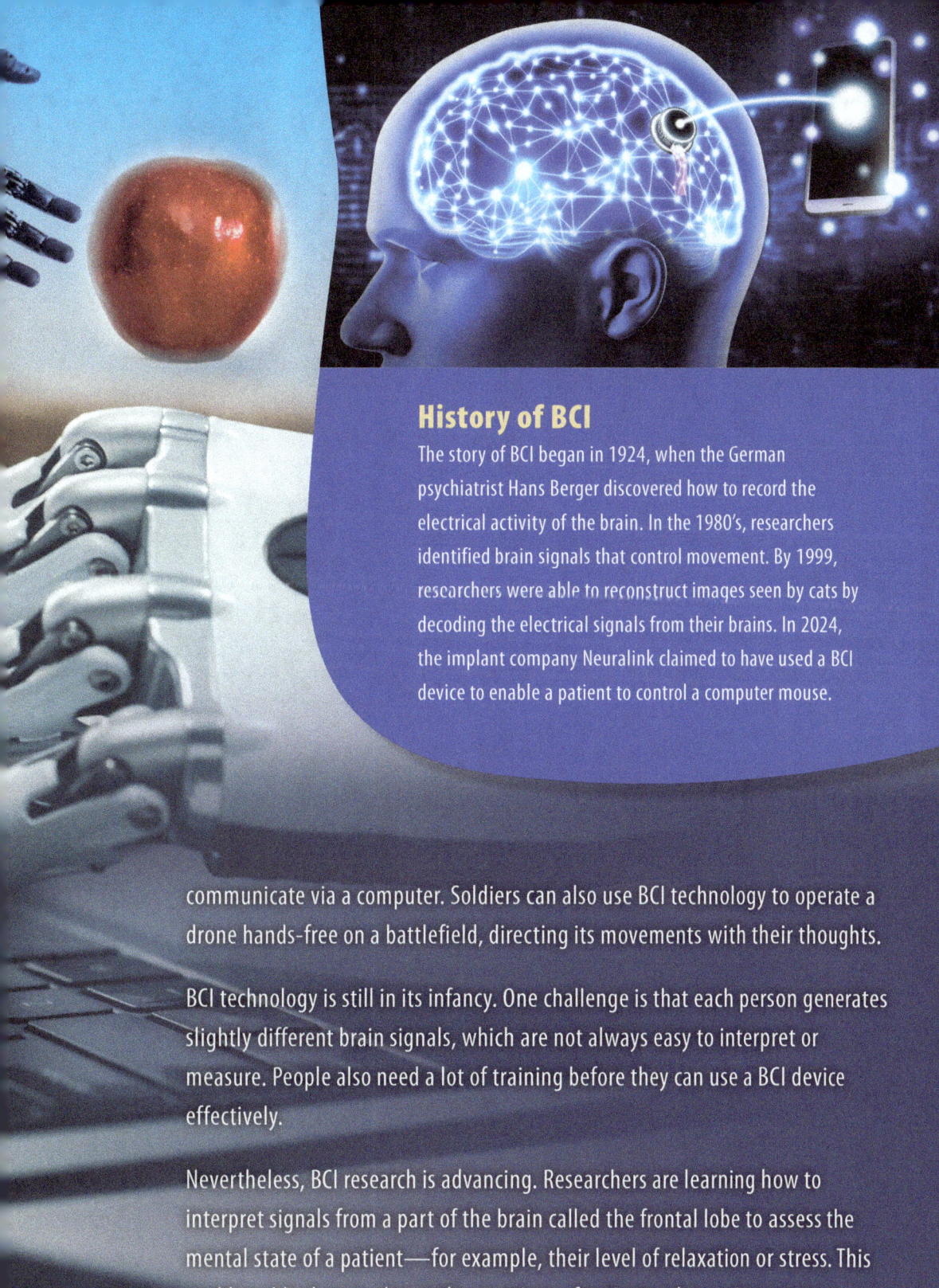

History of BCI

The story of BCI began in 1924, when the German psychiatrist Hans Berger discovered how to record the electrical activity of the brain. In the 1980's, researchers identified brain signals that control movement. By 1999, researchers were able to reconstruct images seen by cats by decoding the electrical signals from their brains. In 2024, the implant company Neuralink claimed to have used a BCI device to enable a patient to control a computer mouse.

communicate via a computer. Soldiers can also use BCI technology to operate a drone hands-free on a battlefield, directing its movements with their thoughts.

BCI technology is still in its infancy. One challenge is that each person generates slightly different brain signals, which are not always easy to interpret or measure. People also need a lot of training before they can use a BCI device effectively.

Nevertheless, BCI research is advancing. Researchers are learning how to interpret signals from a part of the brain called the frontal lobe to assess the mental state of a patient—for example, their level of relaxation or stress. This could enable them to detect the emotions of patients who are in a coma.

Cloned monkeys:
The perfect twins

Two identical long-tailed macaques—named Zhong Zhong and Hua Hua—are the world's first cloned monkeys! They were born in China in 2017. As the first primates to be successfully cloned, the twins represent an important milestone in medical research.

Cloning produces individuals that are genetically identical to each other. This is useful in studying the role of specific genes in disease and other biological processes. Monkeys are more similar to humans than other animals that have been cloned. This makes them valuable for studying how genes might play a role in such human afflictions as Alzheimer's disease.

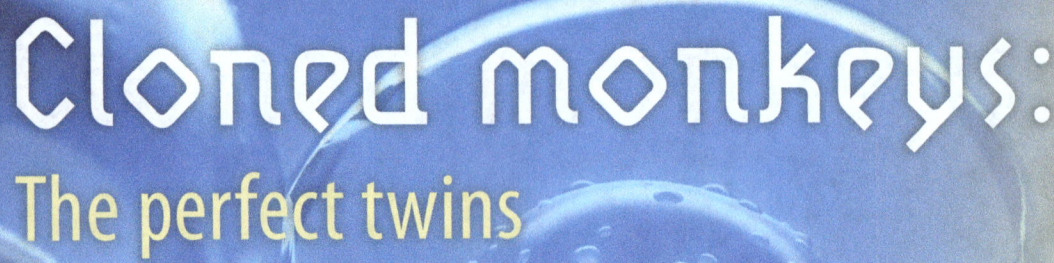

Sheep first
Dolly the sheep, born in 1996, was the world's first cloned mammal. She was cloned using nuclear transfer, a technique that replaces DNA inside an egg cell with DNA from a donor. The result is a genetically identical animal.

Ethical concerns

Scientists have concerns about using monkeys in medical research. Monkeys are genetically similar to humans, and this makes them valuable for research. But they can also experience pain, suffering, fear, and distress, like humans. In the future, advances in technology and research methods may give researchers tools that can replace or reduce the use of live animals.

The scientists who cloned Zhong Zhong and Hua Hua used a method called nuclear transfer. In this process, scientists remove the nucleus from a cell of the animal to be cloned. The nucleus contains the cell's genetic material. Scientists inject the donor nucleus into an egg cell whose own nucleus has been destroyed. The egg cell, with its new nucleus, is genetically identical to the donor animal. Scientists then implant the cloned embryo into the womb of a surrogate (substitute) mother of the same species, who will carry the clone until birth.

Cloning primates is especially complex and difficult. Previous attempts to clone macaques ended with embryos that never became healthy animals. The Chinese team developed several innovative techniques to clone their twin macaques. Still, out of 60 embryos, Zhong Zhong and Hua Hua were the only successful live births.

CLOUD COMPUTING:

Storing data remotely

Have you ever heard the phrase "save it to the cloud"? This makes it sound as though our computer files are being stored in some white, fluffy thing in the sky. It is a nice image, but that is not how cloud computing works.

Cloud computing simply means that data, text files, or software are not stored on your own computer. Instead, you access them over the internet. The files are stored on powerful computers in large data centers all over the world.

You may have used cloud computing without realizing it. When you use a file-sharing service such as Google Drive, Dropbox, or OneDrive, you save your files to the cloud.

Cloud computing has many advantages. It means home and work computers don't need huge memory banks. Data can be stored on a remote database and retrieved only when needed. In the past, damaging your computer might mean losing important files forever. With cloud computing, those files are still safely stored somewhere.

Cloud computing also allows us to access our files on any computer connected to the internet. We can check our emails—or continue working on a project—wherever we are. Software companies use the cloud to send out new versions and fixes to their programs.

All these benefits come with some risks. For example, a power outage can prevent people from accessing the cloud. Another problem is security. Cybercriminals can try to access, destroy, or steal data stored on the cloud.

Protecting the cloud

Cloud computing providers protect data from cybercriminals using encryption. They build firewalls—digital barriers that scan computer traffic to keep malware out. Users must enter a password to access their data. For added security, they might also need to enter a code received by text message.

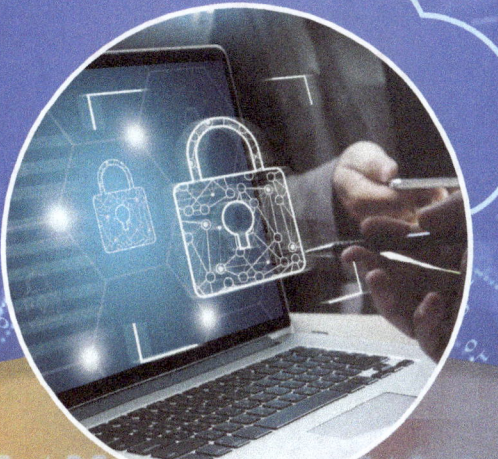

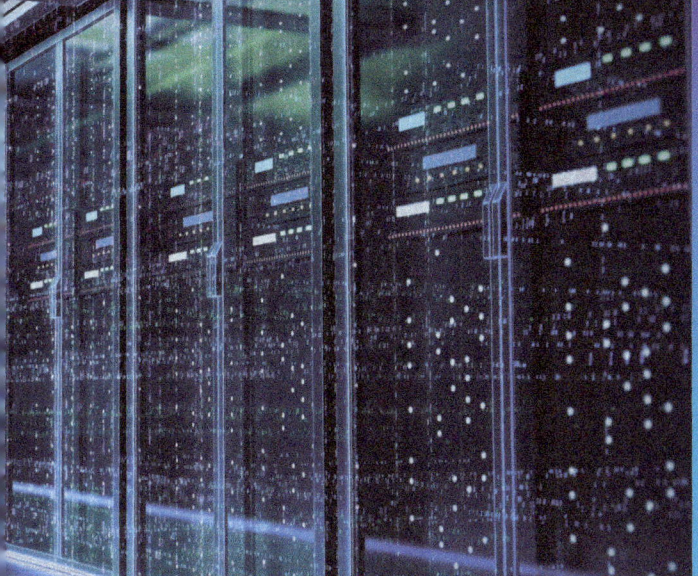

Inventing the cloud

Cloud computing traces its origins to the 1960's, when digital data began to be stored on networks of big computers. The term "cloud" was invented in 1994 by David Hoffman, an employee of American software company General Magic.

CRISPR:
Changing our DNA

Imagine a future where we can alter crops to make them more productive and hardy, or change ourselves to become stronger, healthier, and more intelligent. These are some of the possibilities of a revolutionary new technology known as CRISPR.

CRISPR is a method of gene editing—adding, removing, or altering single genes (sections of DNA) in living cells.

CRISPR is based on the way bacteria and other microbes defend against invading viruses. When infected by a virus, a microbe captures a small piece of the virus's DNA and copies it into its own DNA, allowing the microbe to "remember" the virus. If the virus attacks again, the microbe produces segments of RNA, a molecule like DNA. The RNA segments recognize the virus's DNA and bind to it. Attached to the RNA is an enzyme, which cuts the virus's DNA apart. An enzyme is a substance produced by living things that can cause chemical reactions.

Scientists adapted this defense system to edit DNA. They create a segment of RNA, known as the guide RNA, with a cutting enzyme attached. The guide RNA moves along the strands of DNA until it finds a specific section that it has been programmed to remember. The enzyme then cuts the DNA at this location. Once the DNA has been cut, mutations can be introduced to disable the gene, or new DNA can be added to alter it.

CRISPR gene-editing methods are named for the enzyme they use. The common CRISPR/Cas9 system uses the enzyme Cas9, which is an abbreviation of CRISPR-associated protein 9.

Genes and DNA

Genes are found in every living thing. They are passed from parent to offspring and determine our traits, from the color of our eyes to the diseases we are likely to develop. Genes are sections of DNA, or deoxyribonucleic acid, a two-stranded master instruction molecule found in every cell of the body.

CRISPR

Discovery

In 2012, French scientist Emmanuelle Charpentier and American biochemist Jennifer Doudna isolated components of the CRISPR/Cas9 system in microbes. They modified it to cut DNA molecules at specific sites. They found they could harness Cas9's ability to delete or insert pieces of DNA with amazing precision.

CRISPR could transform medicine, enabling us to treat or prevent many diseases and disorders. Some diseases, such as cystic fibrosis, hemophilia, and sickle cell disease, are caused by genetic mutations. It is now possible, thanks to CRISPR, to insert DNA to fix the mutated genes. Researchers are currently looking at ways of using CRISPR to reprogram immune system cells, so they are able to fight cancer better.

The technology also has applications in farming. Modifying a crop's genes can make it better able to resist disease and tolerate climate change, while also improving its appearance, flavor, and shelf life.

CRISPR could also help improve the health and well-being of farm animals. Researchers in Montevideo, Uruguay, have modified the genes of pigs to make them immune to swine flu. In another experiment, they created a hornless breed of Holstein cattle, because horned cattle are more likely to harm each other.

Better flavor

The American biotech company Pairwise is using CRISPR to reduce the bitterness in leafy salad greens and berries. By improving the flavor of these healthy foods, more people may be encouraged to eat them.

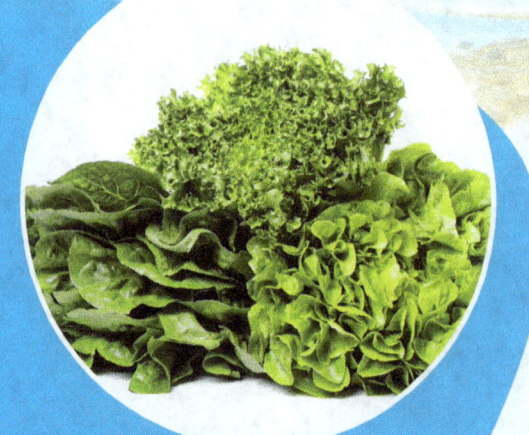

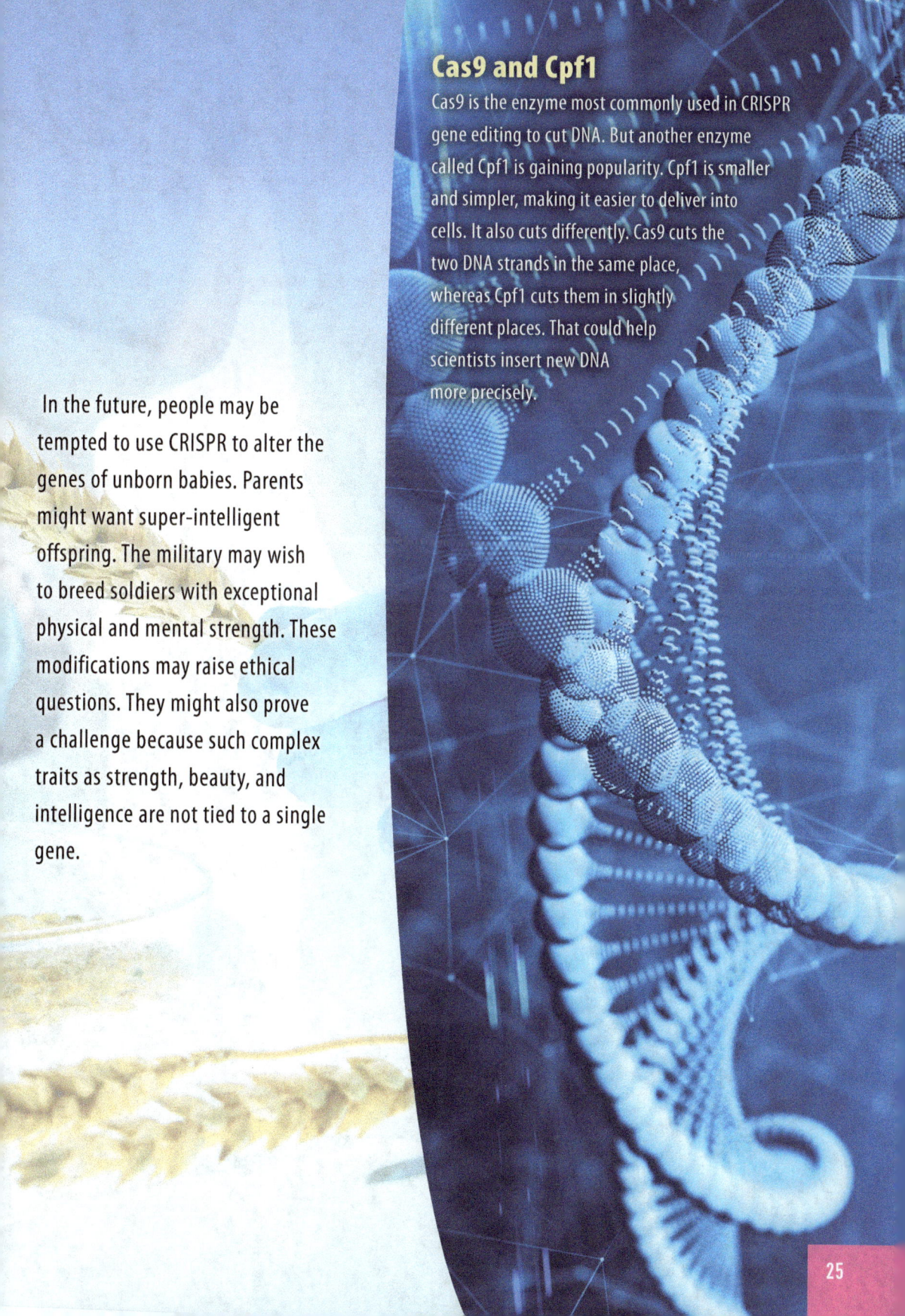

Cas9 and Cpf1

Cas9 is the enzyme most commonly used in CRISPR gene editing to cut DNA. But another enzyme called Cpf1 is gaining popularity. Cpf1 is smaller and simpler, making it easier to deliver into cells. It also cuts differently. Cas9 cuts the two DNA strands in the same place, whereas Cpf1 cuts them in slightly different places. That could help scientists insert new DNA more precisely.

In the future, people may be tempted to use CRISPR to alter the genes of unborn babies. Parents might want super-intelligent offspring. The military may wish to breed soldiers with exceptional physical and mental strength. These modifications may raise ethical questions. They might also prove a challenge because such complex traits as strength, beauty, and intelligence are not tied to a single gene.

CubeSats:
Big science in a tiny package

Thousands of artificial satellites orbit Earth. These devices relay communication signals, monitor the planet's surface, and peer out into space. But traditional satellites are expensive to build and launch—in part because they are so heavy. It costs tens of thousands of dollars to send each kilogram into space. In the early 2000's, a smaller breed of satellite—called the CubeSat—aimed to make a giant dent in the cost of launching.

A CubeSat fits all the parts of a satellite into a small cube, just 10 centimeters (4 inches) on a side, weighing about 1 kilogram (2 pounds). Multiple CubeSats can link to form a larger satellite.

CubeSats are powered by a battery or solar panel. Each also has an antenna to send and receive signals, a small computer, and instruments needed to carry out its mission.

Some CubeSats test materials for use in space. Others photograph Earth or nearby planets. In 2018, the United States launched a

Students in space

The Canadian CubeSat Project gives university students and professors the opportunity to design and build a CubeSat. The first CubeSats from the project launched in 2022.

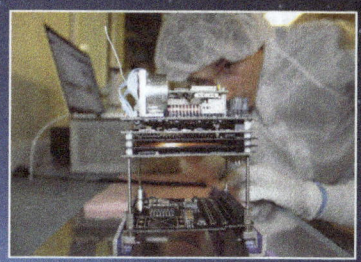

Iconic duo

The MarCO CubeSats were nicknamed WALL-E and EVA, after two robots in the animated motion picture *WALL-E* (2008). Both CubeSats used compressed gas to maneuver in space.

CubeSat mission called Mars Cube One (MarCO for short). Two MarCO CubeSats flew by Mars and sent photographs back to Earth.

The circuits and microchips used to make CubeSats are widely available, similar to those found in smartphones and laptop computers. The CubeSat body is often aluminum, which is cheap and lightweight, although it provides less protection from space-borne radiation than heavier satellite shielding.

Because they are so small and light, CubeSats can be launched in groups. They can also hitch a ride into space with a larger satellite or other launch. When a CubeSat's mission is over, the tiny craft burns up completely on reentering Earth's atmosphere.

EVENT HORIZON TELESCOPE:
The Earth-sized observatory

Imagine a star bigger than our sun being crushed to a tiny point. Think how dense that point would be. If you got close, the gravity would be so powerful that nothing, not even light, could escape. We call these objects black holes, and there are many in our universe.

Because black holes generate no light, they have been hard to spot—until the invention of the Event Horizon Telescope (EHT).

Launched in 2009, the EHT is a network of observatories in different parts of the world that combine their data to act like a single, powerful telescope the size of Earth. This method is known as very-long baseline interferometry (VLBI).

The EHT spots black holes by observing the space around them. All black holes have a boundary, the event horizon, beyond which gravity becomes too strong for anything to escape. With some very large black holes, a disk of glowing gas and dust circles the event horizon. Astronomers call this an accretion disk. It is this glowing disk that the EHT observes.

The EHT project has given us new insights into how matter behaves in extreme gravity. It has created the first photo images of black holes, confirmed Einstein's theory of gravity, helped astronomers estimate a black hole's spin, and spotted a black hole's "shadow" on the accretion disk.

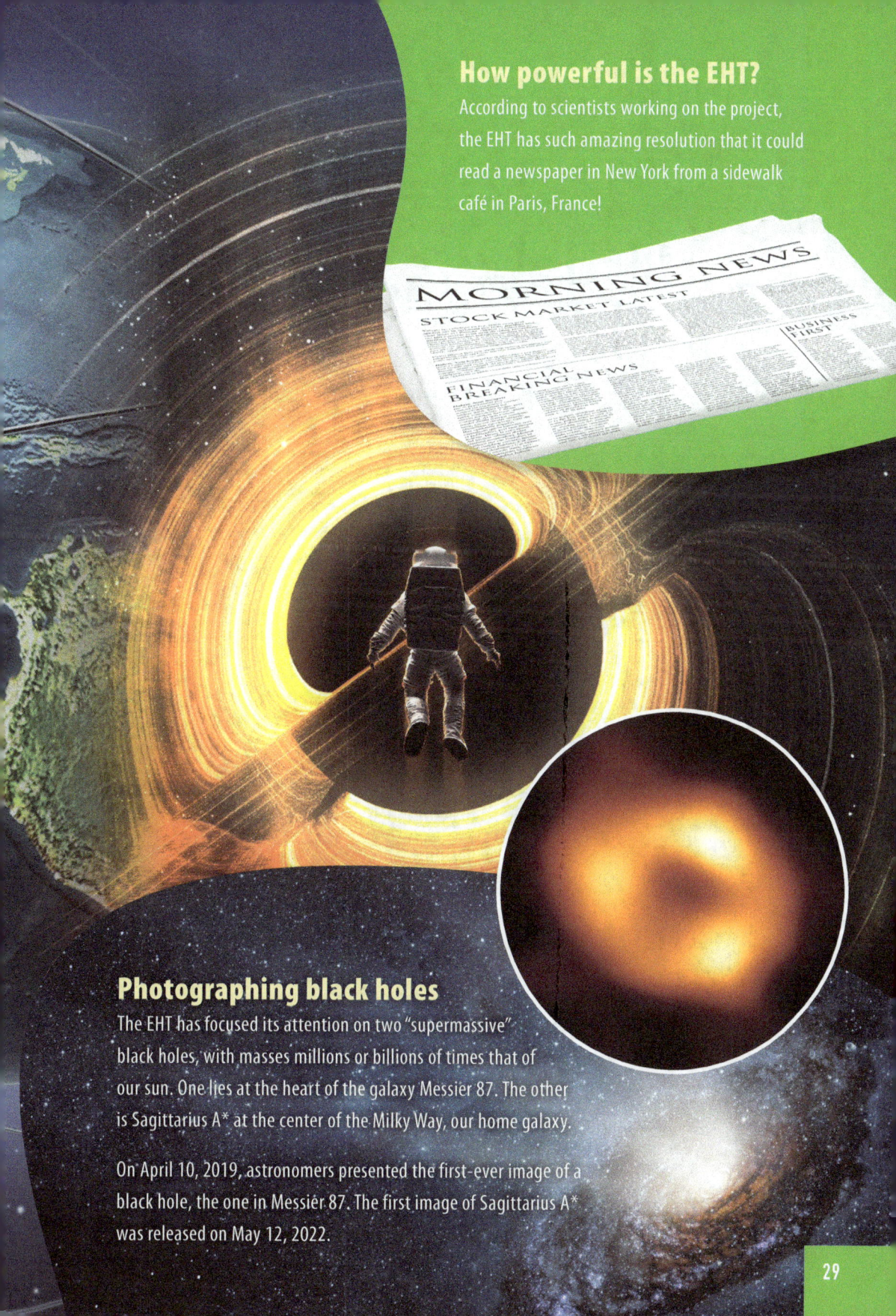

How powerful is the EHT?

According to scientists working on the project, the EHT has such amazing resolution that it could read a newspaper in New York from a sidewalk café in Paris, France!

Photographing black holes

The EHT has focused its attention on two "supermassive" black holes, with masses millions or billions of times that of our sun. One lies at the heart of the galaxy Messier 87. The other is Sagittarius A* at the center of the Milky Way, our home galaxy.

On April 10, 2019, astronomers presented the first-ever image of a black hole, the one in Messier 87. The first image of Sagittarius A* was released on May 12, 2022.

FOODS FROM GENETICALLY MODIFIED ANIMALS:
A customized farm

Genetically modified organisms (GMO's) can be found in any modern grocery store. Most are grains, fruits, and vegetables. But what about meat?

Virtually all foods people consume today come from plants and animals that have been gradually modified through thousands of years of selective breeding by farmers. These species are genetically different from their wild ancestors. Since the 1980's, scientists have used genetic engineering to speed the process up.

Genetic engineering allows us to add, remove, or change an organism's genetic material to produce desirable traits. At first, these techniques were mostly used to tweak plants.

In 2017, a GMO farmed salmon was approved for sale in Canada and later in the United States. Scientists inserted a gene from another fish species that produces growth hormone. The genetically engineered salmon reach market size in 18 months—half the time of traditional farmed or wild salmon. The fast-growing fish help lower production costs and increase the supply of seafood.

In 2020, the U.S. Food and Drug Administration (FDA) approved the genetically modified Galsafe pig for consumption. These pigs do not produce a sugar molecule called alpha-gal. This molecule is naturally found in pigs, but it is absent in humans, where it sometimes causes an allergic reaction to meat.

Frankenfoods

Critics of GM animals often refer to them as "Frankenfoods." The term comes from Mary Shelley's 1818 novel *Frankenstein*, in which a scientist creates a creature using body parts from different people. GM opponents argue that genetic engineering uses genes from unrelated species in ways that are unpredictable and potentially harmful.

In 2022, the FDA approved genetically engineered cattle called PRLR-SLICK. These cattle have short hair and are more heat-tolerant. This helps the cattle avoid heat stress, which can harm their health and reduce their weight.

Today, only a few genetically modified animals have been approved for commercial use. But we may soon see more.

No need for a flu shot

Researchers are engineering animals so they are immune to avian influenza, a deadly bird disease that sometimes spreads to farm animals—especially chickens and ducks. However, GM opponents believe avian influenza is better controlled through better farming practices rather than genetically engineering disease-resistant chickens.

HOLOGRAMS:
3D images that move

You may have seen holograms in movies—3D images that can move around in the real world and even talk. Simple holograms can be found all around us, printed on driver's licenses and credit cards. But what exactly are holograms?

Holograms are created by splitting a laser beam in two. One beam reflects off the object you want to photograph and onto a high-resolution film or photographic plate. The other beam shines directly onto the film. Where these two light beams cross on the film, they make a complex, microscopic pattern of bright and dark stripes called an interference pattern.

When light shines on the hologram, the interference pattern changes the direction of bounced light so that the light rays appear to come from the original illuminated object. The resulting three-dimensional image seems to hover in space. When you move around it, you can view it from different angles, and sometimes the color changes. It has *motion parallax* (things in the foreground move faster than things in the background), and you see two different images with each eye, giving the impression of depth.

Some companies are experimenting with holograms in virtual reality headsets. Paired with sensors that track a user's eyes and hand movements, they could make virtual objects feel more real.

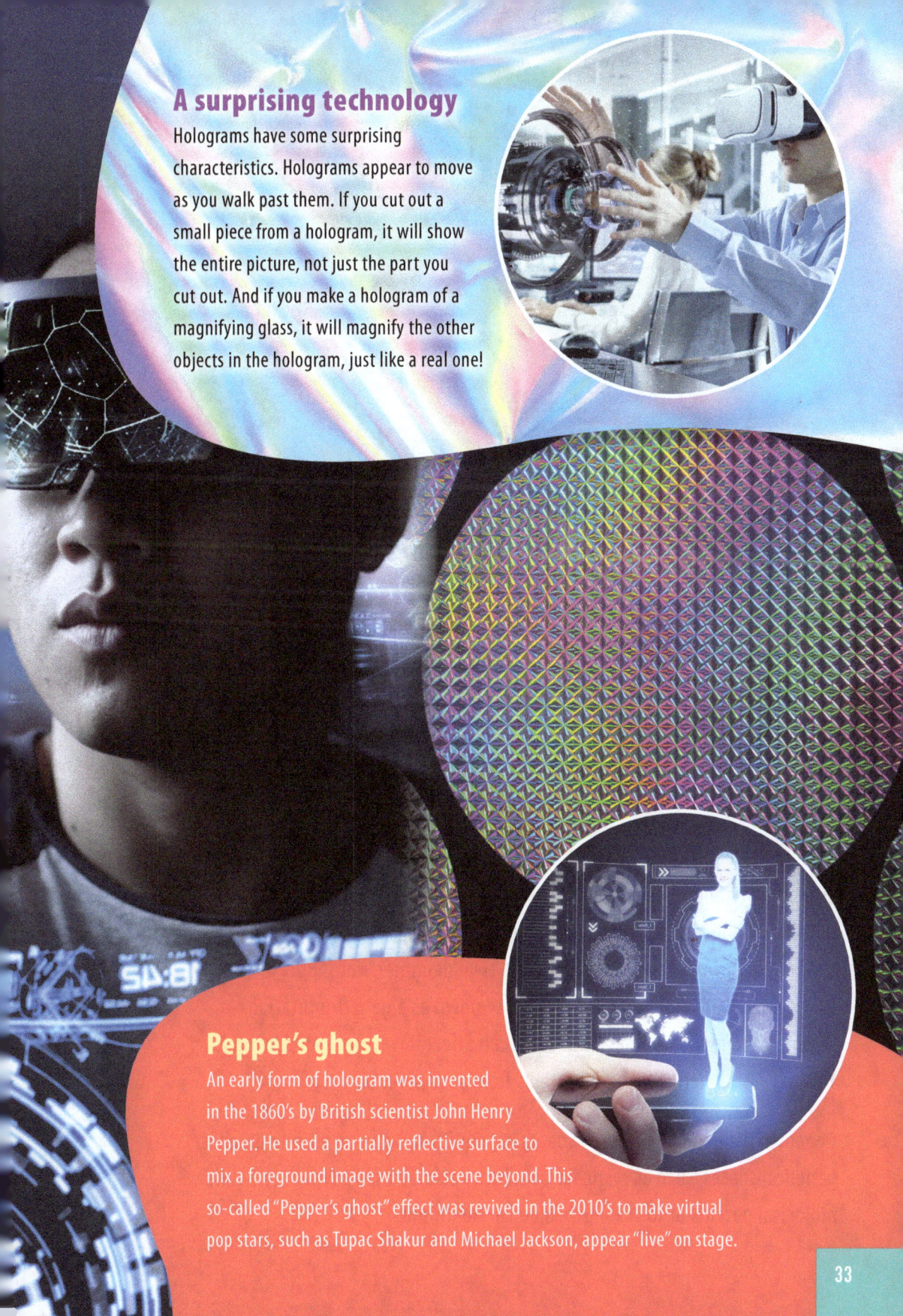

A surprising technology

Holograms have some surprising characteristics. Holograms appear to move as you walk past them. If you cut out a small piece from a hologram, it will show the entire picture, not just the part you cut out. And if you make a hologram of a magnifying glass, it will magnify the other objects in the hologram, just like a real one!

Pepper's ghost

An early form of hologram was invented in the 1860's by British scientist John Henry Pepper. He used a partially reflective surface to mix a foreground image with the scene beyond. This so-called "Pepper's ghost" effect was revived in the 2010's to make virtual pop stars, such as Tupac Shakur and Michael Jackson, appear "live" on stage.

HOME GENETIC TESTING:

Predicting health risks

Today, you can mail some of your spit to a company, and a few weeks later they will tell you whether you are likely to go bald or what part of the world your ancestors came from. Since home genetic testing began in 2007, millions of people have taken these tests to find out more about themselves.

Genetic testing tests your DNA—the substance that makes up your genes (see facing page). The same set of DNA is found in almost every cell in your body. When a cell divides, the DNA inside it is copied to the two "daughter" cells. But sometimes there is a copying error. This is known as a genetic mutation. Most mutations are harmless, but some can affect how your body functions. You may also inherit genetic mutations from your parents.

Genetic testing looks for gene variants in your DNA. It can be used to diagnose genetic diseases, such as cystic fibrosis. It can also be used to identify a child's biological parents or to customize medical treatments.

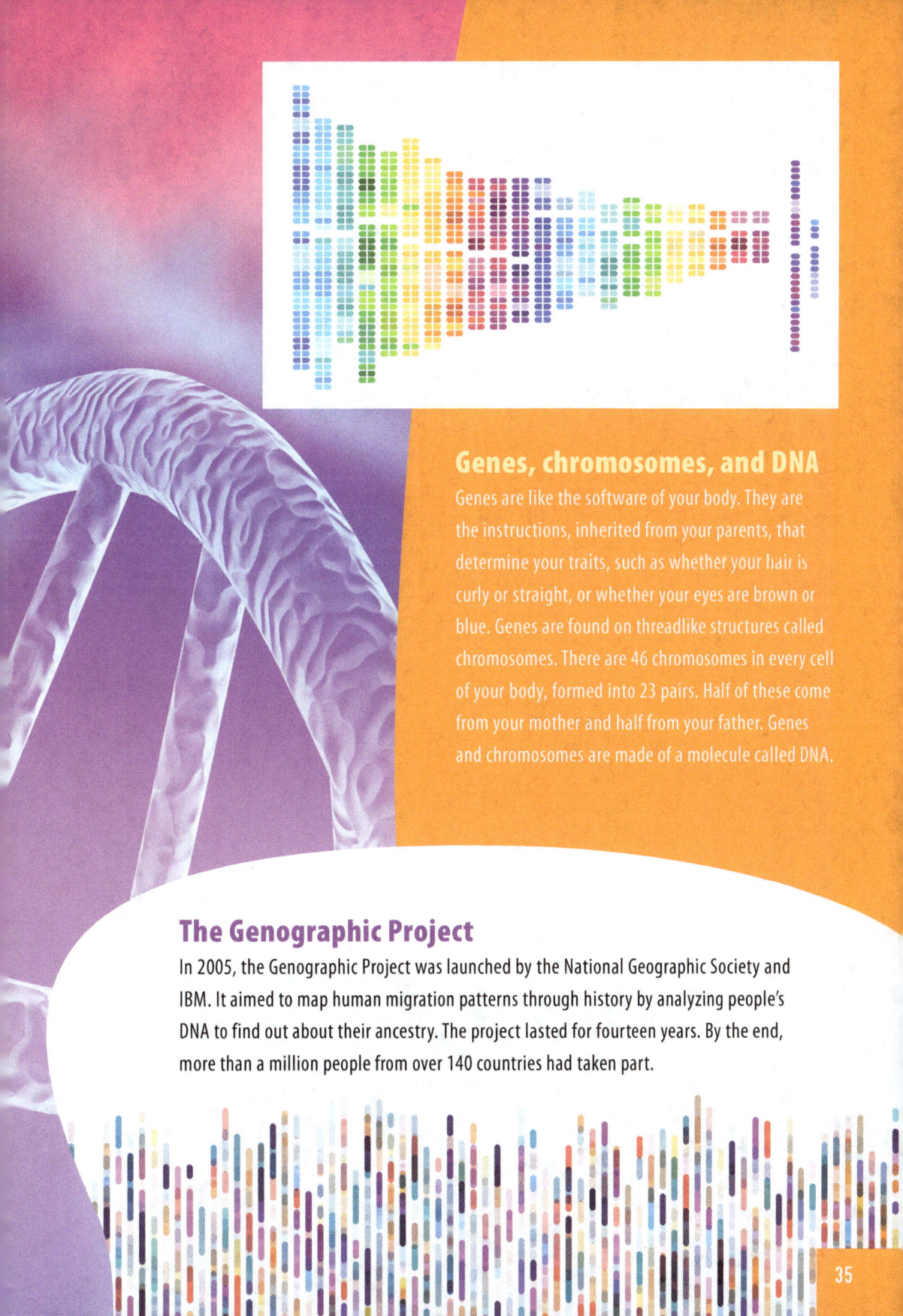

Genes, chromosomes, and DNA

Genes are like the software of your body. They are the instructions, inherited from your parents, that determine your traits, such as whether your hair is curly or straight, or whether your eyes are brown or blue. Genes are found on threadlike structures called chromosomes. There are 46 chromosomes in every cell of your body, formed into 23 pairs. Half of these come from your mother and half from your father. Genes and chromosomes are made of a molecule called DNA.

The Genographic Project

In 2005, the Genographic Project was launched by the National Geographic Society and IBM. It aimed to map human migration patterns through history by analyzing people's DNA to find out about their ancestry. The project lasted for fourteen years. By the end, more than a million people from over 140 countries had taken part.

Home genetic tests to determine ancestry are especially popular. These compare the DNA variants in an individual with DNA variants common in populations from different geographic regions across the world.

Companies offering home genetic testing services require a sample of the customer's DNA. This could be in the form of saliva, blood, or cells collected from the inside of the cheek (a cheek swab). Once the company's laboratory receives the sample, the DNA is extracted from it. First it is amplified (see facing page), then it is cut into small pieces and placed on a *microarray chip*, a small glass plate encased in plastic.

Each microarray chip contains the DNA sequence of thousands of normal genes and some common mutations. When an individual's DNA sample is added to the chip, it binds to the DNA already there. Genes with mutations will not bind to normal genes, but will bind to matching variants.

Home genetic testing can be a quick, simple way to get information about one's health and risk of disease. However, it is also important to get advice from a healthcare professional. Genetic tests can only provide part of the picture. Environmental factors and lifestyle choices also have a big influence on our health.

DNA sequencing

Genes are made of DNA, which contains four chemicals called bases: adenine (A), cytosine (C), thymine (T), and guanine (G). In every gene, these four bases arrange themselves in different ways. Working out the order of these bases is known as DNA sequencing. Every gene has its own DNA sequence.

Amplifying a DNA sample

For a good genetic test, companies like to have a large sample of DNA. When they get your drop of spit, they first extract the DNA and amplify it, or make millions of copies. DNA is made up of two long strands twisted around each other. In a technique called a polymerase chain reaction (PCR), laboratories first untwist the strands with heat. Then they add a polymerase enzyme, which binds to the DNA and builds two identical new strands. New molecules of DNA form, composed of one old and one new strand of DNA. Then these are separated into two strands again, and the cycle repeats. After 35 to 40 rounds, there are millions of identical copies of the original DNA sample.

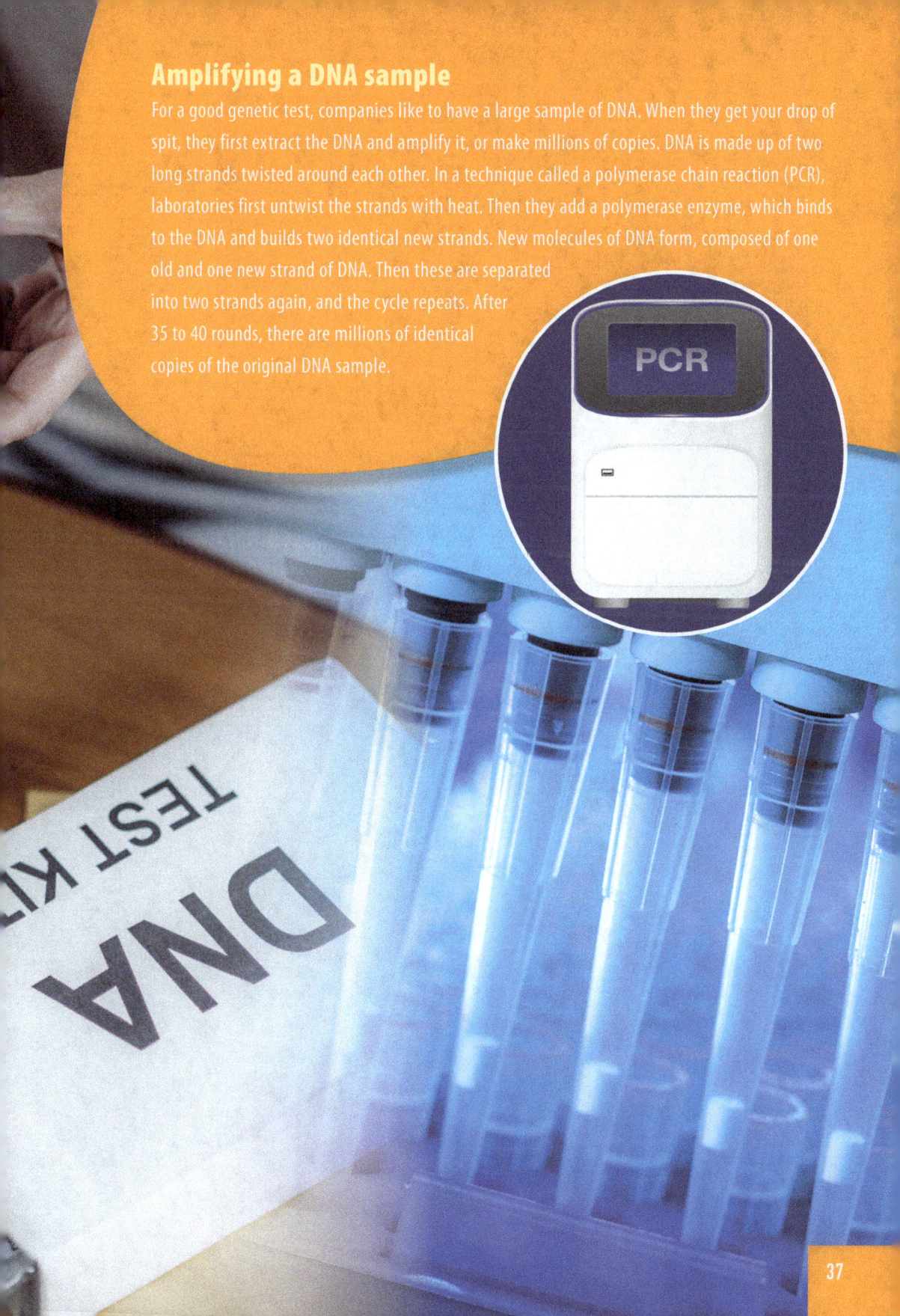

HUMAN GENOME:
Learning about ourselves

Imagine being given a medicine that is perfectly tailored to you as an individual. Today, this is becoming possible thanks to advances in the field of human genomics.

Genomics is the study of the genome—the complete set of genes in an organism. Genes are sections of DNA that produce traits (see p. 35). They are passed from parent to offspring.

DNA is arranged in two twisting strands. Each strand is made up of long strings of "bases," which come in four types, called A, T, G, and C for short. Each base links with one on the opposite strand. Working out the order of bases in DNA is known as sequencing.

The Human Genome Project (HGP), launched in 1990, set out to sequence the entire human genome. That's approximately 3.1 billion base pairs, so it was an ambitious goal! The project cost billions of dollars and involved thousands of researchers around the world.

In one of the great achievements in scientific history, the HGP reached its goal in 2003, sequencing 92 percent of the human genome. The final 8 percent was sequenced by 2022.

The HGP opened the way for many innovations in healthcare. It has helped scientists better understand how genes affect such diseases as cancer, diabetes, and high blood pressure.

The HGP took 13 years, but today an individual's genome can be sequenced in a matter of hours. Checking a patient's genome helps doctors assess risks for certain diseases so they can provide preventative treatments. It can also help them predict how a patient may respond to particular medicines or other treatments.

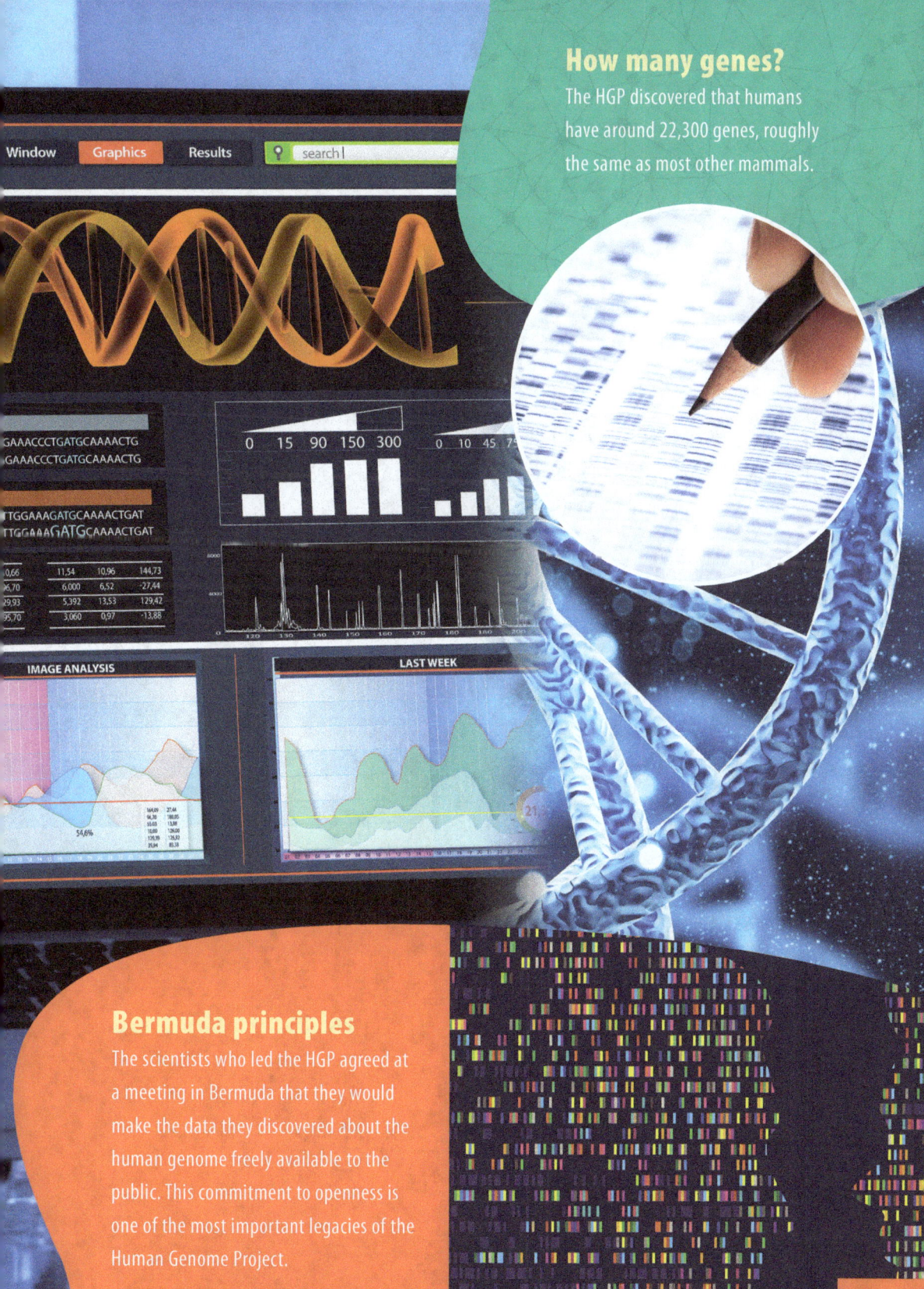

How many genes?

The HGP discovered that humans have around 22,300 genes, roughly the same as most other mammals.

Bermuda principles

The scientists who led the HGP agreed at a meeting in Bermuda that they would make the data they discovered about the human genome freely available to the public. This commitment to openness is one of the most important legacies of the Human Genome Project.

Infrared thermometer:
The "temperature gun"

One of the biggest problems in fighting a contagious illness is figuring out who is sick. Fever can be an important sign of infection. Unfortunately, we cannot tell who is hot just by looking. We can, however, measure temperature at a glance using an infrared thermometer.

The infrared thermometer has been nicknamed the "temperature gun" because it is held the same way. The end facing the patient holds a sensor and sometimes a laser to help aim. A display screen provides a readout of the target's temperature. A compartment in between holds electronics.

Infrared thermometers were first developed during the mid-1900's but came into widespread use around 2000, when parts used to make them became smaller and cheaper.

Infrared thermometers were widely used during the COVID-19 *pandemic* (worldwide outbreak) that began in 2019. They allowed health professionals to quickly screen people for fever with minimal contact.

Infrared thermometers work by measuring infrared radiation, an invisible light that objects give off as atoms move around. Hotter objects are brighter in infrared. In an infrared thermometer, a sensor called a thermopile converts incoming infrared radiation into an electrical signal. A computer converts that into a temperature, which is displayed on a small screen.

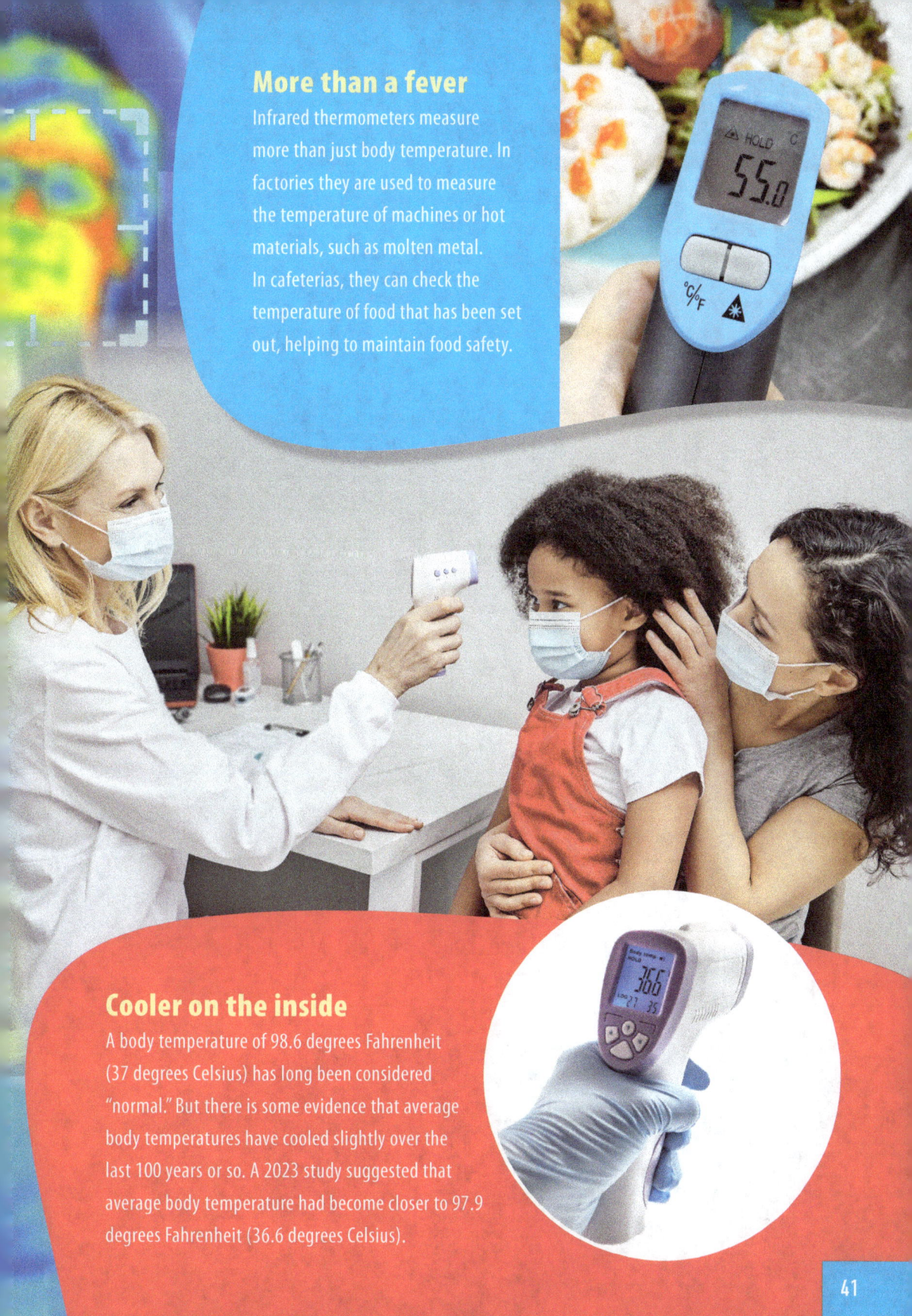

More than a fever

Infrared thermometers measure more than just body temperature. In factories they are used to measure the temperature of machines or hot materials, such as molten metal. In cafeterias, they can check the temperature of food that has been set out, helping to maintain food safety.

Cooler on the inside

A body temperature of 98.6 degrees Fahrenheit (37 degrees Celsius) has long been considered "normal." But there is some evidence that average body temperatures have cooled slightly over the last 100 years or so. A 2023 study suggested that average body temperature had become closer to 97.9 degrees Fahrenheit (36.6 degrees Celsius).

JAMES WEBB SPACE TELESCOPE:
Looking back at the early universe

Far from Earth, a giant space observatory watches the universe, sending us images of ancient galaxies and distant planets. NASA's James Webb Space Telescope (JWST) is the largest and most powerful space telescope ever built.

Launched in December 2021, the JWST orbits the sun, around 930,000 miles (1.5 million kilometers) from Earth. The JWST collects infrared light, which we can't see but can feel as heat. Infrared light is not blocked by space dust. That means the JWST can see through dust clouds to witness the formation of stars and planets. It can also see very distant objects such as the first galaxies, which are moving away from us so fast that their light is stretched out into the infrared part of the spectrum. The JWST can also see such faint objects as planets that would normally be obscured by the brightness of their star.

To detect faint infrared signals from distant objects, the JWST must be kept extremely cold. A gigantic five-layer sun shield the size of a tennis court stays between the JWST and the sun. Thanks to the sun shield, the infrared instruments are kept at temperatures as low as -447 °F (-266 °C).

Orbit

The JWST orbits the sun at a point in space called the L2 Lagrange point. This keeps the telescope in line with Earth, so astronomers can remain in constant communication and download images from the telescope.

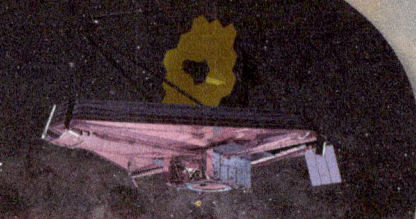

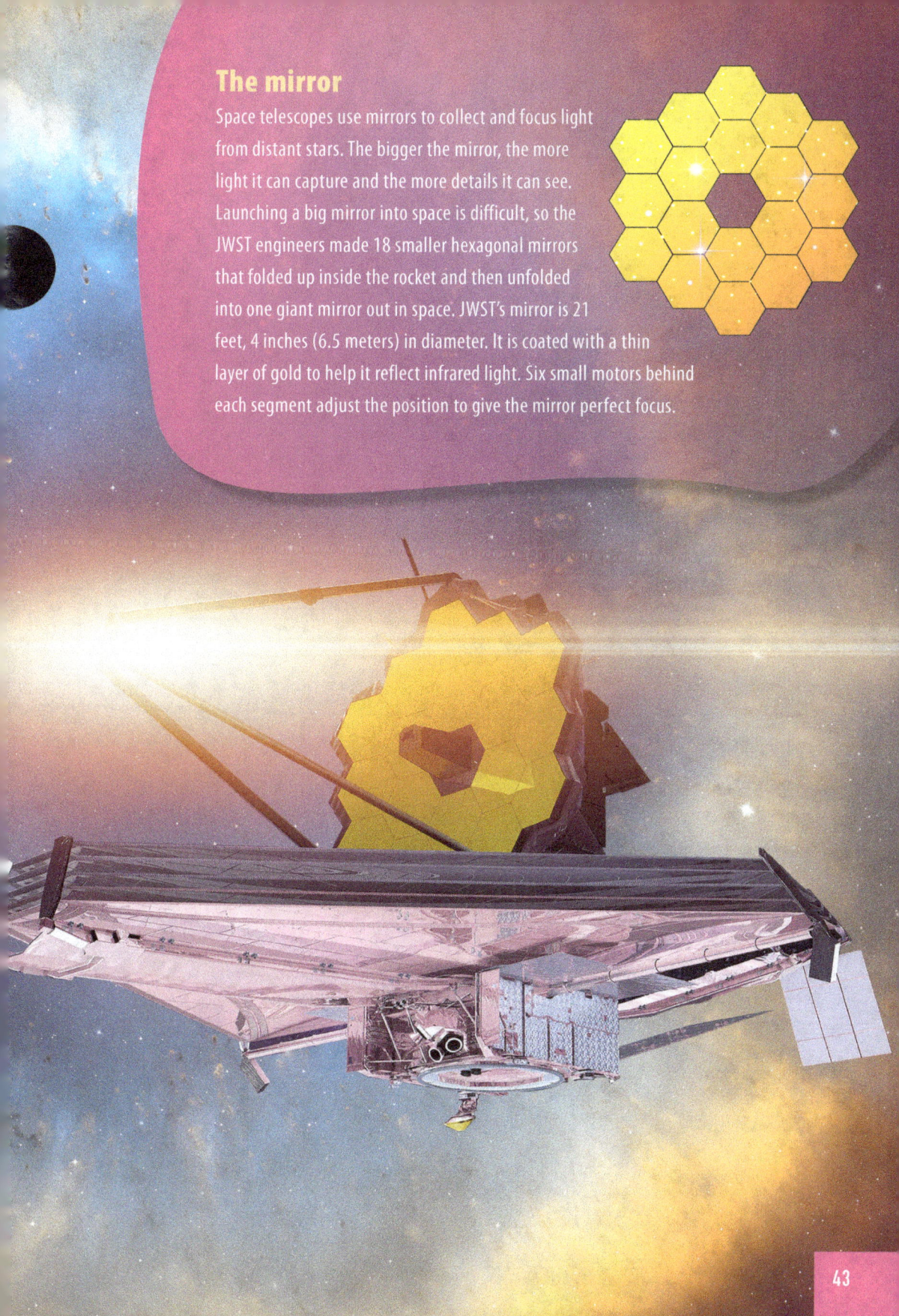

The mirror

Space telescopes use mirrors to collect and focus light from distant stars. The bigger the mirror, the more light it can capture and the more details it can see. Launching a big mirror into space is difficult, so the JWST engineers made 18 smaller hexagonal mirrors that folded up inside the rocket and then unfolded into one giant mirror out in space. JWST's mirror is 21 feet, 4 inches (6.5 meters) in diameter. It is coated with a thin layer of gold to help it reflect infrared light. Six small motors behind each segment adjust the position to give the mirror perfect focus.

As well as an infrared camera, the JWST is equipped with an infrared spectrograph. This tool spreads out the light it captures into a spectrum, showing all the wavelengths and their intensity. This can reveal the chemical composition of the atmospheres of planets, which might reveal the presence of life.

In September 2023, the JWST's spectrograph detected carbon dioxide on Jupiter's moon Europa. We already know that Europa has water, a key ingredient of life. The discovery of carbon dioxide increases the chance that microbial life could exist there. The JWST also spotted carbon dioxide and methane in the atmosphere of K2-18b, a planet in another solar system about 120 light-years from Earth. This raises the possibility that life could exist in other parts of the universe.

When we gaze at the night sky, we are looking back in time. It can take millions or billions of years for the light from the stars we see to reach our eyes. Therefore, we are seeing how those stars appeared in the distant past. With its powerful mirror and infrared vision, the JWST can peer back in time over 13.5 billion years, to the very first stars and galaxies that formed shortly after the *big bang*, when our universe began. By comparing the galaxies of the early universe to the spiral and elliptical galaxies of today, astronomers can start to understand how galaxies assemble and evolve over billions of years.

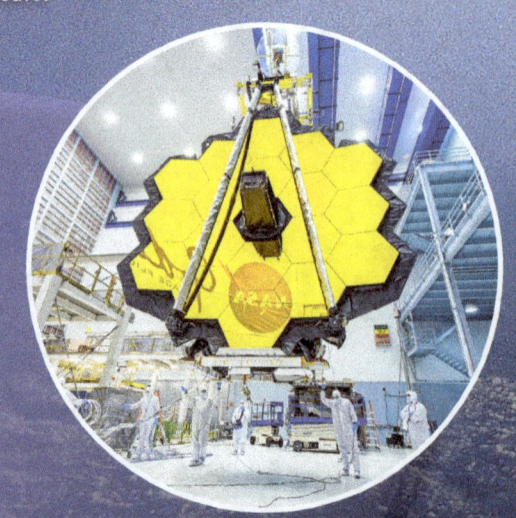

Launch and deployment

JWST was launched on December 25, 2021, and arrived at its destination on January 24, 2022. It then required several months to align its mirrors to create a single primary mirror. On July 11, 2022, the telescope captured its first scientific image, which showed the deepest-ever infrared view of the universe. It took 12.5 hours of observation time to create.

James Webb

The JWST is named for former NASA chief James Webb, who led the space agency from 1961 to 1968 during the first part of the Apollo moon program. Under Webb's leadership, NASA launched more than 75 space missions.

Redshift

Because the universe is constantly expanding, the light coming to us from distant stars and galaxies shifts to longer wavelengths at the redder end of the spectrum. This is known as redshift. Observing infrared allows astronomers to study this light in better detail, increasing their understanding of the earliest stars and galaxies.

LAB-GROWN MEAT:
From laboratory to table

Food scientists have long sought meat alternatives that look and taste like the real deal without the need to raise and slaughter animals. But many people feel that soy patties and mushroom burgers just aren't the same. Now, there is a new cruelty-free way to get real meat—grow it in a lab!

The process of creating real meat in a laboratory without animals is pretty straightforward. Scientists take a sample of cells from a chicken or cow. From that sample, scientists create an "immortalized" cell line, one that can be kept alive indefinitely. Next, the cells are "fed" a mixture of amino acids, fatty acids, vitamins, and minerals. Cells and food are placed in a cultivator—a sterile metal container that's heated, pressurized, and oxygenated. After about a month, the meat can be harvested. Meat from a lab tends to be a bit paler, but otherwise, it looks and tastes the same as meat from an animal.

There are many benefits to lab-grown meat. On a modern farm, livestock need shelter, space to roam, food, healthcare, and transportation. Animals also take time to mature. Lab-grown meat can be produced continuously on an industrial scale. It releases fewer greenhouse gases and takes up less space. That means it might be able to feed more people for the same cost.

At the moment, lab-grown meat is still very expensive. The first lab-grown hamburger cost $330,000 to make in 2013. A pound (0.5 kilogram) of lab-grown beef costs around $17 to produce today. But experts expect the cost to go down as the technology improves.

Lab-grown Meat

FUTURE OF PROT[EIN]

Cooking instructions
Grill or pan fry for half minutes side at medium heat. Season to your taste and they are delicious

PLEASE DO NOT OVER COOK

Robotic taste test

To taste the first samples of lab-grown meat, researchers used an electronic tongue made up of multiple sensors. They found that changing what the cells are fed gives the lab-grown meat different qualities.

Safer food

Because lab-grown meat is produced in a sterile environment, the meat is less likely to be contaminated with such food-borne germs as salmonella or *E. coli* bacteria.

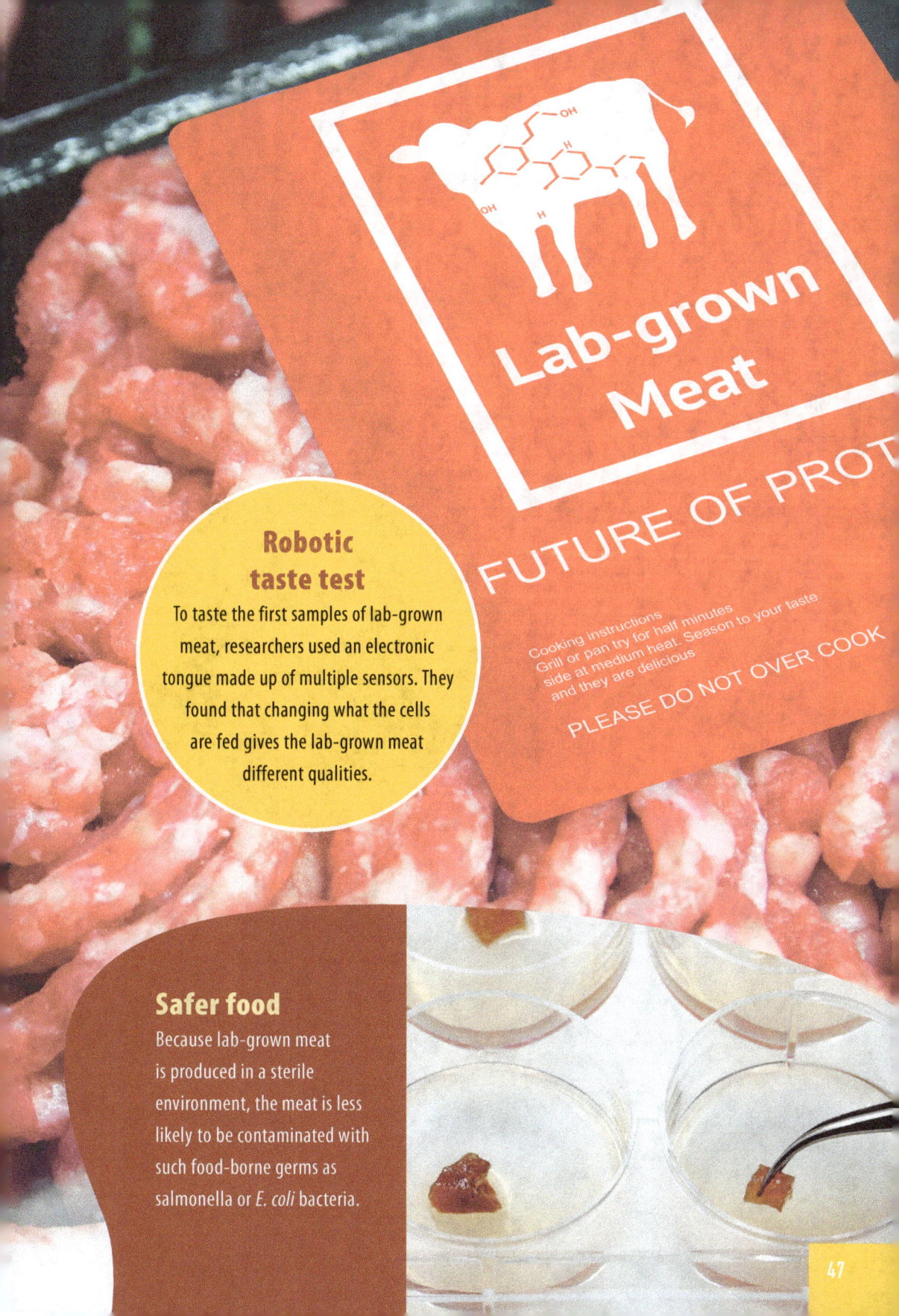

Large HADRON COLLIDER:
Uncovering the secrets of the universe

Imagine accelerating particles to 99.99 percent of the speed of light and then smashing them together. That is the job of the Large Hadron Collider (LHC).

The LHC is a *particle accelerator*—a machine that propels tiny subatomic particles, such as protons or electrons, at close to the speed of light, smashing them into a target or against other particles. Studying the collisions helps physicists learn more about the nature of matter and the universe's origins.

The LHC is the world's largest and most powerful particle accelerator. It is a giant circular tube, 17 miles (27 kilometers) in circumference, built beneath the French-Swiss border by CERN (the European Organization for Nuclear Research). More than 8,000 scientists from 60 different countries work there.

When an experiment is run, first all air is removed from the tube. Then particles are accelerated by 9,300 powerful magnets. They race around the LHC ring 11,245 times a second, resulting in millions of particle collisions.

Physicists use the LHC to test the predictions of the Standard Model. According to this model, everything in the universe is made from a set of fundamental particles governed by four forces. Physicists hope the LHC can help answer some big questions, such as why gravity is weaker than the other forces. The LHC might also help to identify dark matter, the mysterious, invisible stuff that might make up more than 80 percent of the universe.

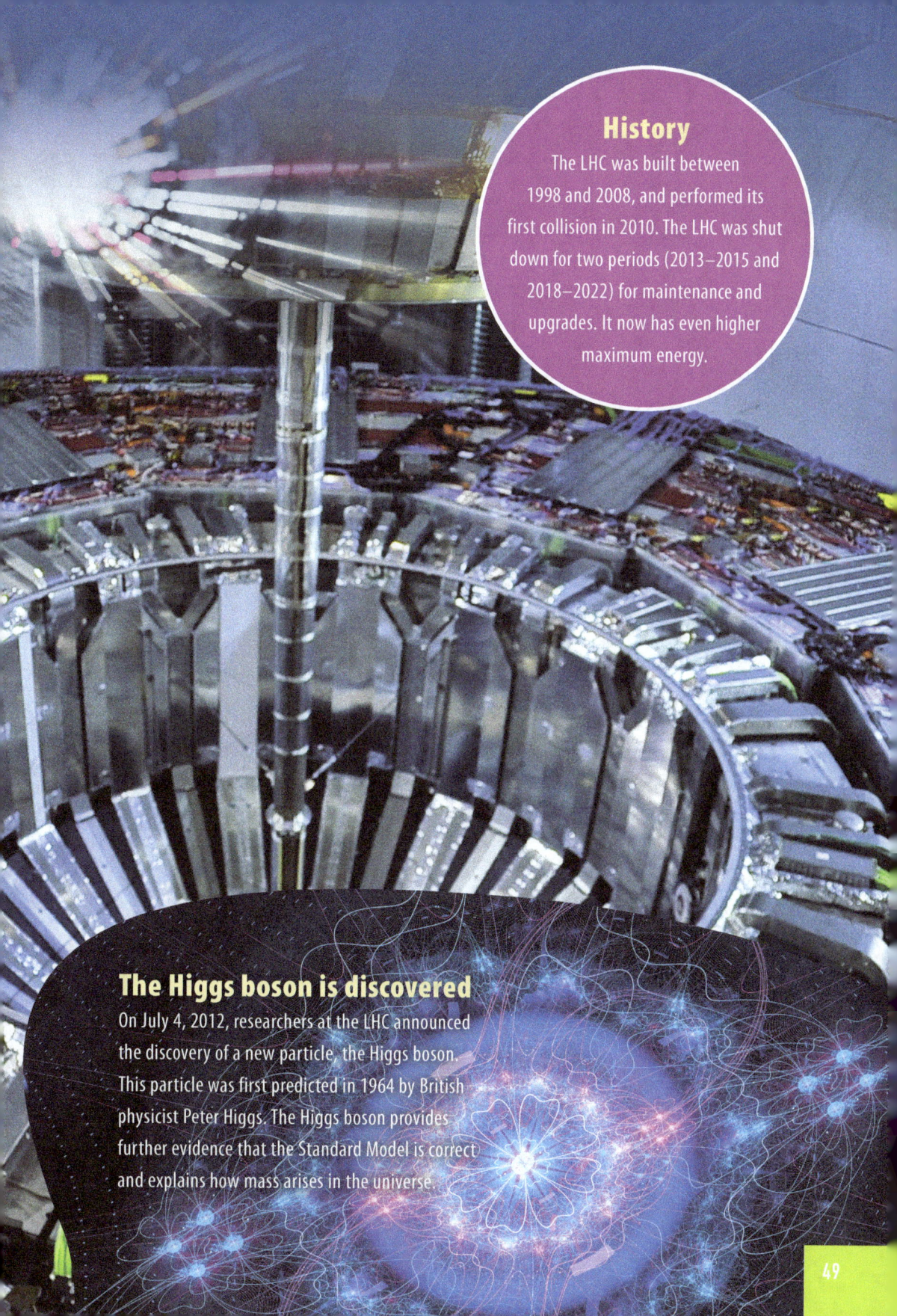

History

The LHC was built between 1998 and 2008, and performed its first collision in 2010. The LHC was shut down for two periods (2013–2015 and 2018–2022) for maintenance and upgrades. It now has even higher maximum energy.

The Higgs boson is discovered

On July 4, 2012, researchers at the LHC announced the discovery of a new particle, the Higgs boson. This particle was first predicted in 1964 by British physicist Peter Higgs. The Higgs boson provides further evidence that the Standard Model is correct and explains how mass arises in the universe.

Laser Interferometer Gravitational-Wave Observatory (LIGO):

Listening to the universe

Massive cosmic events, such as colliding and exploding stars, send ripples through space known as gravitational waves. By the time these reach Earth, they are extremely weak. The ripples may be ten thousand times smaller than the nucleus of an atom! Could a device be built to detect something so tiny? The answer is yes, and the device is the Laser Interferometer Gravitational-Wave Observatory, or LIGO.

LIGO consists of two detectors 1,864 miles (3,000 kilometers) apart, operating together. Each detector is shaped like an L. The two arms are vacuum tubes 2.5 miles (4 kilometers) long, with mirrors at either end. Gravitational waves cause tiny changes in the lengths of the arms. These changes are detected by laser beams bouncing between the mirrors.

Super sensitive

At its most sensitive, LIGO will be able to detect a gravitational wave 1/10,000th the width of a proton—the smallest measurement ever attempted in the history of science. It is equivalent to measuring the distance to the nearest star (about 25.2 trillion miles, or 37.8 trillion kilometers away) to an accuracy smaller than the width of a human hair.

Gravitational waves

The physicist Albert Einstein predicted the existence of gravitational waves in 1916. His equations showed that giant cosmic events would send ripples out through space in all directions. In 1974, astronomers found the first evidence in two stars orbiting each other. The stars were moving closer together at the exact rate predicted if they were emitting gravitational waves.

LIGO was built in the 1990's and started looking for gravitational waves in 2002. On September 14, 2015, it caught one, caused by the collision of two black holes 1.3 billion light years away.

As technology improves, LIGO's detectors will become ever more sensitive. Gravitational waves can improve our understanding of the cosmos and maybe gravity itself. In the words of Argentinian physicist Gabriela González, they allow us to "hear the universe."

Earth's curvature

LIGO's arms are so long that the Earth curves away by nearly a meter over their length. The contour of the concrete path on which they were laid had to be adjusted to allow for this, so the laser beams could travel in a straight line.

METAMATERIALS:
Turn yourself invisible

Have you ever wanted an invisibility cloak, so you can walk around undetected? It may become possible thanks to metamaterials. These are artificial materials with special surfaces that manipulate light and other forms of energy.

Metamaterials are not made of any special kind of substance. It's their physical structure that gives them their unique properties. At very small scales, their atoms and molecules are arranged into geometric patterns, like a lattice. This allows them to interact with light in ways that are not found in nature.

Because of their structure, metamaterials can *refract* (bend) light. This can make it look a different color. A sheet of gold with a metamaterial surface might appear red or green, although the gold itself has not changed. Metamaterials could also bend the paths of light waves around an object, a bit like a boulder diverting water in a stream. Someone looking at the object would see what's behind it, while the object itself would be invisible. This type of metamaterial might someday be used to create an invisibility cloak.

A metamaterial with a structure that captures light from a wide range of angles might help solar cells collect more sunlight, with less light reflected, or wasted. Metamaterials that reduce unwanted reflected light could also improve the lenses of cameras, telescopes, and glasses.

Sound effects

Imagine a material that could make sounds louder or softer. Some metamaterials have a structure that can manipulate sound rather than light energy. They could be designed to amplify or reduce sound waves or focus them in a particular direction.

Metasurfaces

Metamaterials are sometimes manufactured as very thin films known as metasurfaces. They can *diffract* (split) light into different numbers of rays and send them out at different angles, depending on the structure of the lattice. Stealth aircraft could one day be coated with a metasurface that makes them invisible to radar (a system used to detect objects using radio waves).

mRNA VACCINES:
Manufacturing immunity

Nobody likes to get a shot—ouch! But some shots can help your body fight disease. These shots are called *vaccines*. They train the body's immune system to fight illness.

Once you have had a contagious illness, you may be less likely to get it again. This is because your immune system "remembers" germs it has fought in the past. It can quickly manufacture chemicals called *antibodies* to fight those germs.

A traditional vaccine works like a fake infection. The vaccine contains inactive germs or germ material. The body's immune cells hunt down and destroy the injected material, just as they would a live infection. The body learns to fight the disease, becoming immune to the real thing.

Traditional vaccines are quite safe. But new mRNA vaccines help your body develop immunity without injecting an actual germ.

mRNA is a molecule that living cells use to make proteins. Proteins are materials that help the cell to do its work. Think of mRNA as something like a blueprint for making a particular protein. The cell's machinery uses the mRNA to manufacture the protein.

mRNA vaccines borrow the cell machinery to make their own proteins. The vaccine mRNA contains instructions for making proteins that sit on the surface of germs. These proteins are just parts of germs—they cannot make you sick. But they can teach the immune system to recognize a germ.

mRNA is short for messenger RNA. It was discovered back in the 1960's. The first widely used mRNA vaccines were developed in 2020 to fight the worldwide outbreak of COVID-19.

Scrambled genes?

Some people worried that mRNA vaccines might "scramble" the body's *genes*. Genes are the instructions for making a living thing. They are encoded in a molecule called DNA. But vaccine mRNA cannot enter the cell *nucleus* (center). This is where the DNA is kept.

Katalin Karikó,

a Hungarian-born American scientist, made important contributions to the development of mRNA vaccines. She helped to figure out how to safely deliver mRNA to the body's cells.

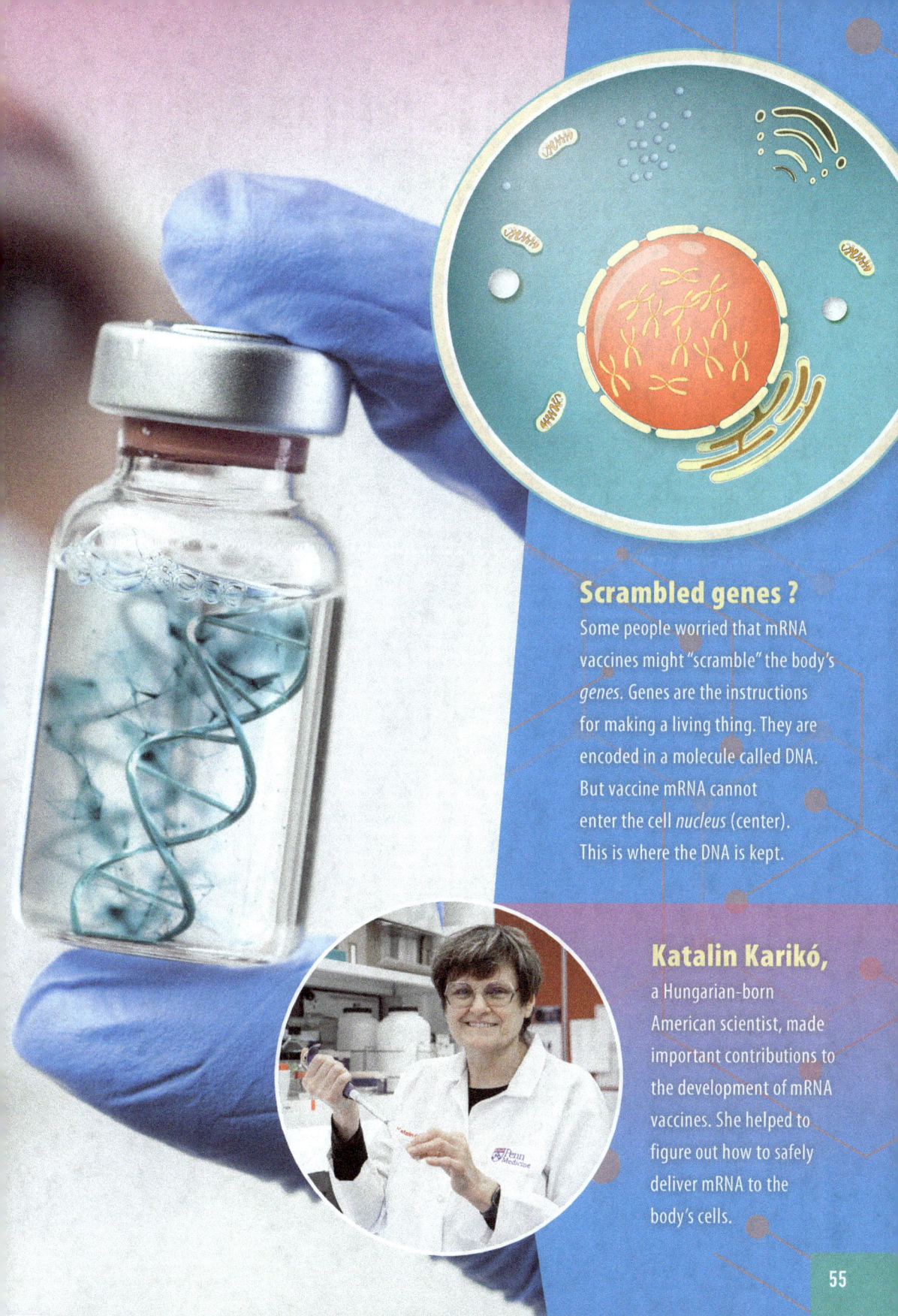

Personal insulin pump:
Life-saving diabetes help in a pod

More than 400 million people around the world live with diabetes. Their bodies either cannot make the hormone insulin or have become less sensitive to it. These people rely on regular injections of insulin to keep them alive and healthy. In the 2000's, a small, wearable insulin pump was invented. This pump—sometimes called a *pod*—sticks directly to the skin and delivers life-saving insulin.

Our bodies get a sugar called glucose from the food we eat. Glucose provides energy for the body's activities. But too much or too little glucose in the blood can have deadly consequences. Normally, the body produces just the right amount of insulin to keep glucose in balance. But people with diabetes have to monitor their blood carefully to avoid problems. When blood glucose gets too high, they must inject insulin to bring it back in line.

For many years, people with diabetes tracked blood glucose by pricking a finger to let a drop of blood fall onto a blood analyzer. Then they gave themselves a shot of insulin if necessary, or pressed a button to deliver insulin through an implanted tube. This meant constant checking and a lot of shots!

The first tubeless system, called Omnipod, was released in 2005. The "pod" looks a bit like a plastic bottle cap attached to a sticker. It sticks to the skin, usually on the upper arm, thigh, lower back, or belly. Underneath the pod is a tiny needle that administers insulin.

Insulin-delivery pods connect wirelessly to smartphones or other devices. They are often used with a continuous glucose monitor (CGM), a wearable device that tracks blood glucose levels all the time. Together, these enable users to enjoy life without worrying about their glucose.

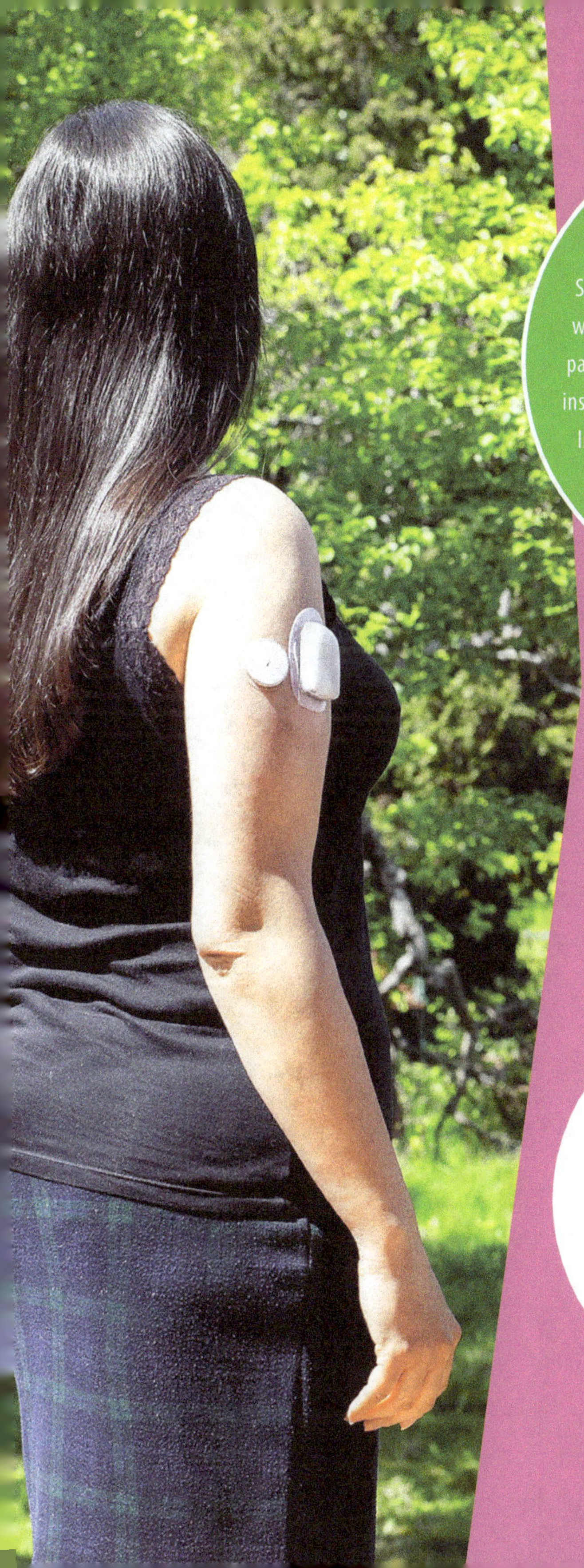

Fashion accessory

Sales of insulin pumps skyrocketed in 1998 when Nicole Johnson won the Miss America pageant. Johnson had daringly displayed her insulin pump in the bathing suit competition. In 2021, the British model Lila Grace Moss Hack wore her Omnipod on the fashion runway, causing a similar stir!

Keep it sticky

To help keep the Omnipod stuck on, Omnipod-shaped stickers come in a variety of fun designs, from unicorns to beloved television characters!

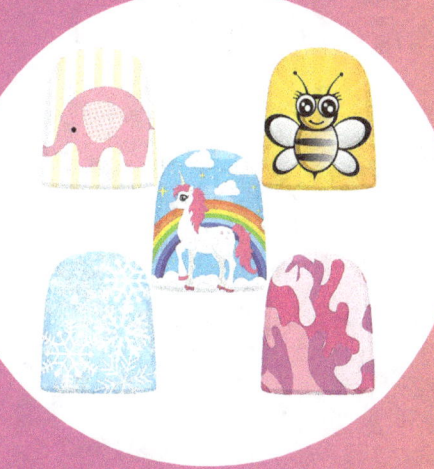

PROSTHETICS:
Helping people move and feel

When people lose limbs or have a limb disability, sometimes they use a replacement called a prosthesis. Early prosthetic legs and arms were simple mechanisms. Today, thanks to advances in engineering, prostheses offer more control, dexterity, and even a sense of touch.

How can a prosthetic hand offer a sense of touch? Sensors in the fingers are connected to electrodes in the arm muscles, which send signals to a computer port in the wearer's skull. The computer passes signals to the sensory part of the brain. Users report a "tingling sensation" rather than a full sense of touch, but it helps them work out how hard to grip something.

Brain-computer interface technology (see page 16) is also allowing people to control the motion of the prosthesis by thinking. Prosthetic devices that respond to signals from the brain are called myoelectric prostheses.

To operate a myoelectric arm, the wearer simply thinks of moving it. This sends brain signals to the muscles in the residual limb. The signals will vary depending on what motion the wearer intends. The muscles contract, generating electric signals. These are detected by electrodes on the skin inside the socket, which send them to a computer in the prosthetic arm. This triggers motors inside the arm to move it in the desired way.

Two-way communication

For a prosthesis to mimic the feel of a biological limb, it needs to communicate with the brain. Ideally, the limb should be able to receive and respond to the brain's commands, and also send information back about how the limb is moving and sensing. Today's myoelectric prostheses can do this. They are equipped with electronic sensors that send feedback to electrodes in the residual limb, which is then relayed through the usual neural pathways to the brain.

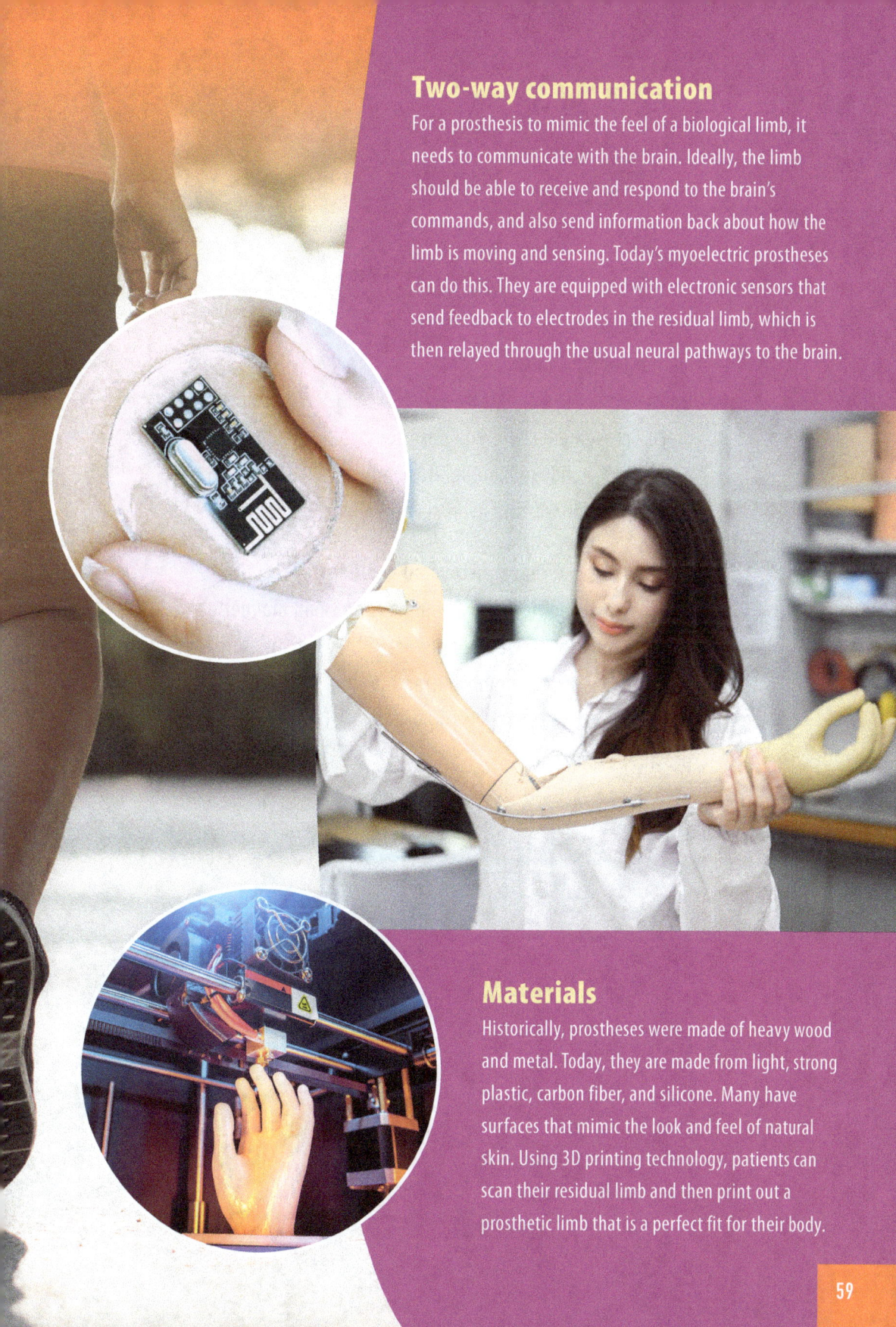

Materials

Historically, prostheses were made of heavy wood and metal. Today, they are made from light, strong plastic, carbon fiber, and silicone. Many have surfaces that mimic the look and feel of natural skin. Using 3D printing technology, patients can scan their residual limb and then print out a prosthetic limb that is a perfect fit for their body.

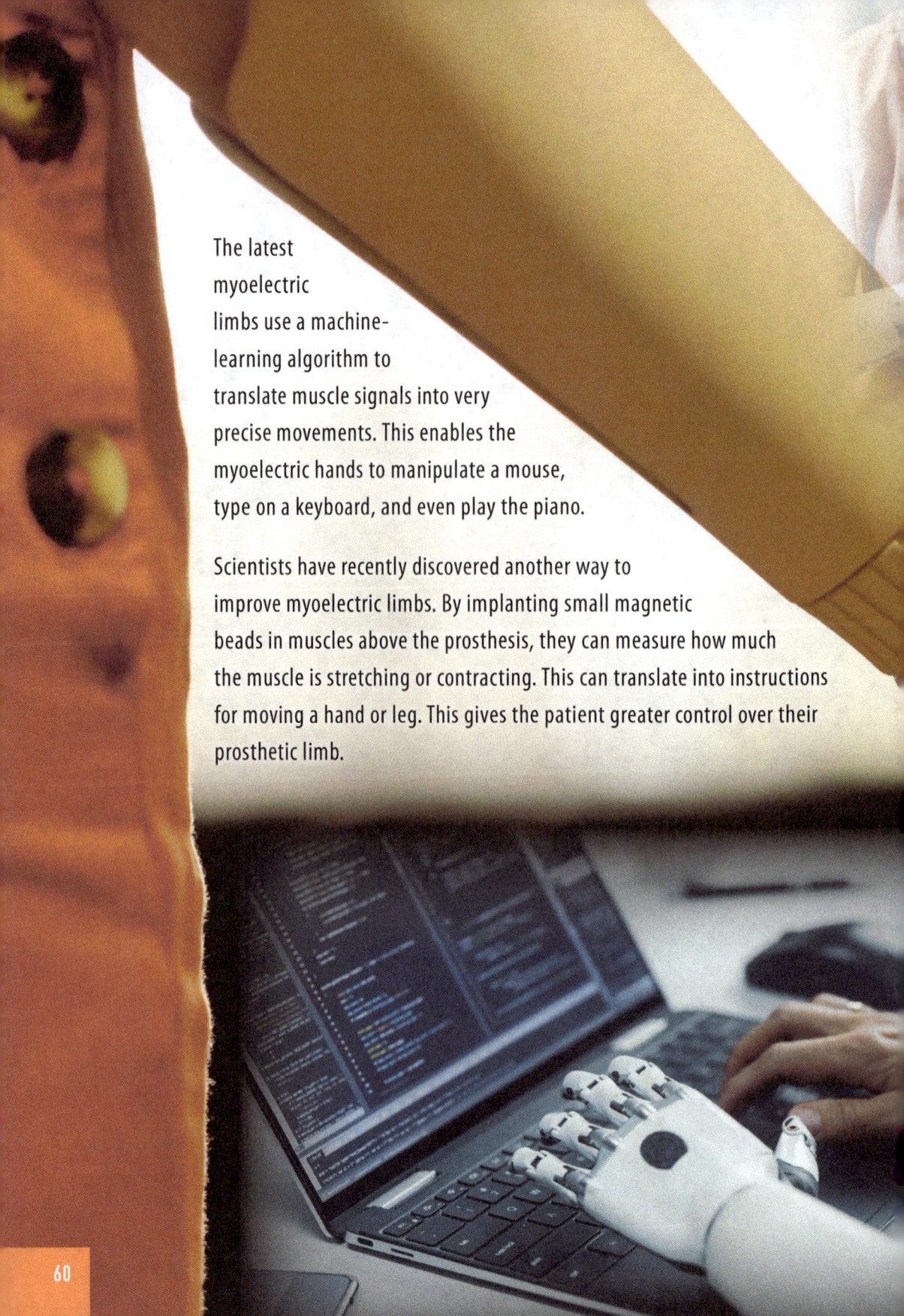

The latest myoelectric limbs use a machine-learning algorithm to translate muscle signals into very precise movements. This enables the myoelectric hands to manipulate a mouse, type on a keyboard, and even play the piano.

Scientists have recently discovered another way to improve myoelectric limbs. By implanting small magnetic beads in muscles above the prosthesis, they can measure how much the muscle is stretching or contracting. This can translate into instructions for moving a hand or leg. This gives the patient greater control over their prosthetic limb.

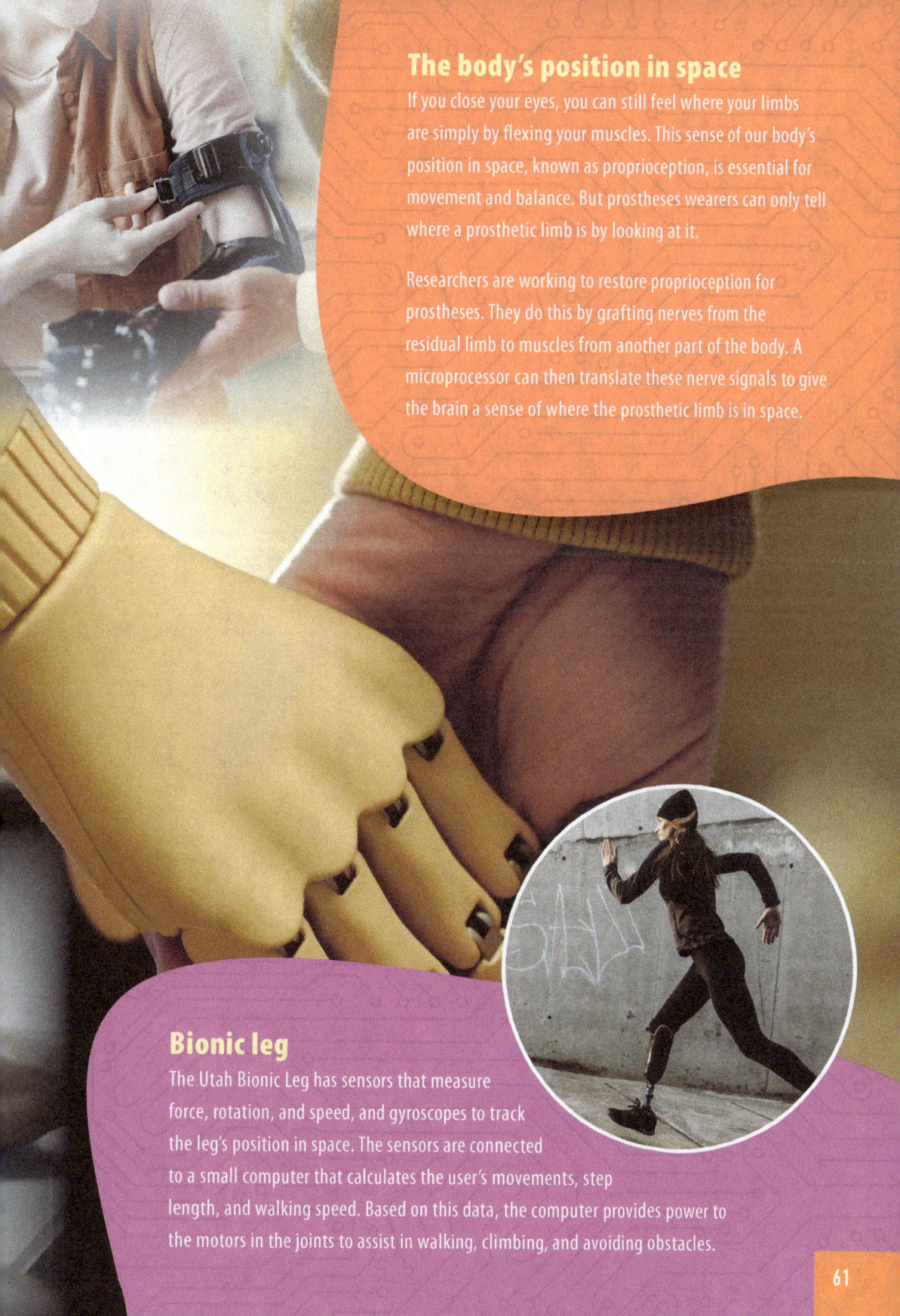

The body's position in space

If you close your eyes, you can still feel where your limbs are simply by flexing your muscles. This sense of our body's position in space, known as proprioception, is essential for movement and balance. But prostheses wearers can only tell where a prosthetic limb is by looking at it.

Researchers are working to restore proprioception for prostheses. They do this by grafting nerves from the residual limb to muscles from another part of the body. A microprocessor can then translate these nerve signals to give the brain a sense of where the prosthetic limb is in space.

Bionic leg

The Utah Bionic Leg has sensors that measure force, rotation, and speed, and gyroscopes to track the leg's position in space. The sensors are connected to a small computer that calculates the user's movements, step length, and walking speed. Based on this data, the computer provides power to the motors in the joints to assist in walking, climbing, and avoiding obstacles.

QUANTUM COMPUTING:
Superfast problem solvers

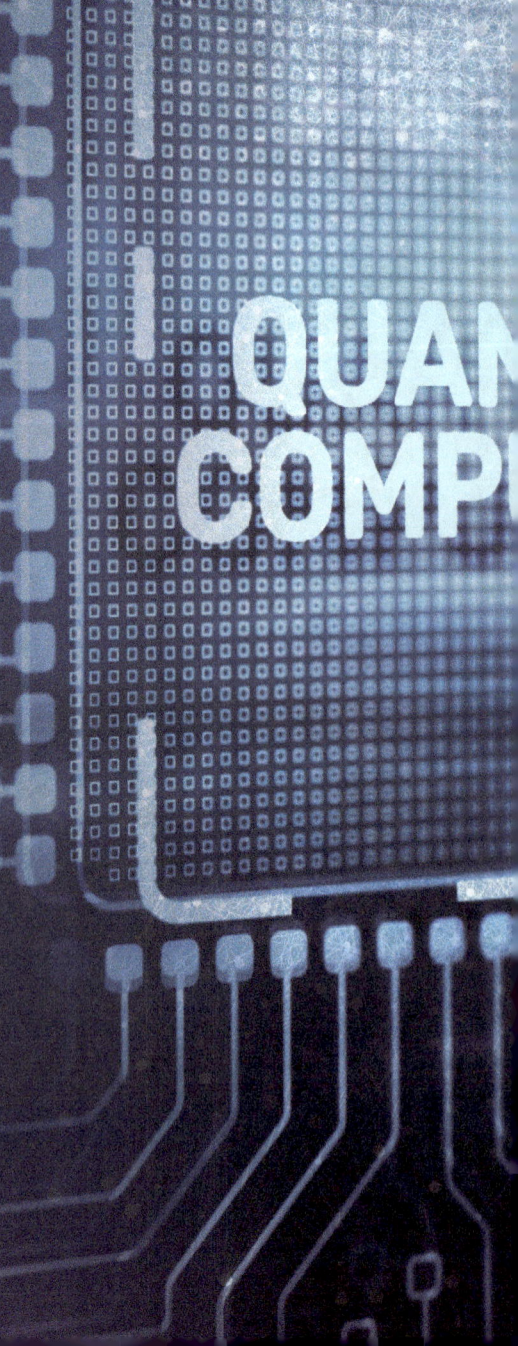

Today's computers may seem pretty fast, but they are positively slothlike compared to a revolutionary new method of computing now being developed. Quantum computing harnesses the special properties of subatomic particles, such as electrons and photons, to solve complex problems thousands of times faster than a classical computer.

Quantum computing excels at problems with many *variables* (elements that are likely to vary or change), such as forecasting the weather or the stock market, developing safer forms of encryption, or modeling the behavior of molecules. How does it do it?

Classical computers encode information using ones and zeros, known as binary digits, or bits. Quantum computers use quantum bits, or qubits. While classical bits are limited to two possible states (one or zero), qubits can be one, zero, or one *and* zero at the same time (known as a superposition).

The fact that qubits have three possible states helps quantum computers solve extremely complex, multidimensional problems.

Quantum particles can also become entangled, meaning two particles are linked even if they are far apart. If a change is made to one particle, the other particle also changes. Entanglement enables qubits to interact instantaneously, increasing a quantum computer's processing power.

Quantum computers for the public may still be some way off. This is because qubits must be kept very cold and not touch any other particles or magnetic fields. That can get expensive. However, quantum computers could soon be used by such large organizations as the military, banks, or medical research institutions.

Decoherence

One problem with quantum computing is decoherence. This happens when qubits decay and fall out of superposition, causing errors in computing. To prevent decoherence, quantum computer processors must be kept super cold—at about a hundredth of a degree above absolute zero.

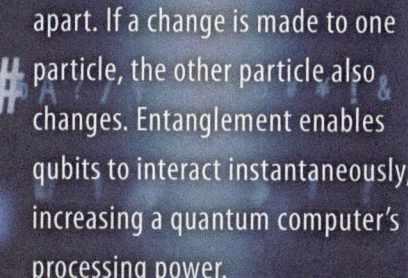

A milestone

In 2019, a quantum computer solved a problem in 200 seconds that would have taken a classical computer approximately 10,000 years to solve.

Retinal implants:
An eye-opening invention

Many people fear blindness more than any other disability. But medical researchers are finding new ways to help.

Retinal implants are a new tool to restore vision. The retina is the innermost layer of the wall of the eyeball. Its sensitive cells (called rods and cones) absorb light rays and send electrical signals to the brain, which the brain interprets as vision. Other cells in the retina help identify images. Retinal implants help people whose retinas have been damaged.

The first successful retinal implant, called the Argus II, was invented in 2011 and approved in the United States in 2013. It is named after Argus, the many-eyed giant from Greek mythology.

The Argus II implant is designed to restore some sight to people who have lost their vision due to retinitis pigmentosa, a disease of the retina. A surgeon implants an electronic device on the retina. A video camera in a pair of eyeglasses transmits images to a portable video processing unit (VPU). The processor then sends signals to the implant.

The implant works by using a small electrode array to stimulate damaged retinal cells. The implant receives visual signals from the VPU. The image triggers electrodes, which activate retinal cells to send visual signals through the optic nerve to the brain.

Eye surgery

A retinal implant is a delicate surgical procedure that takes 1.5 to 4 hours. Surgeons must perform several tests to make sure the device works correctly.

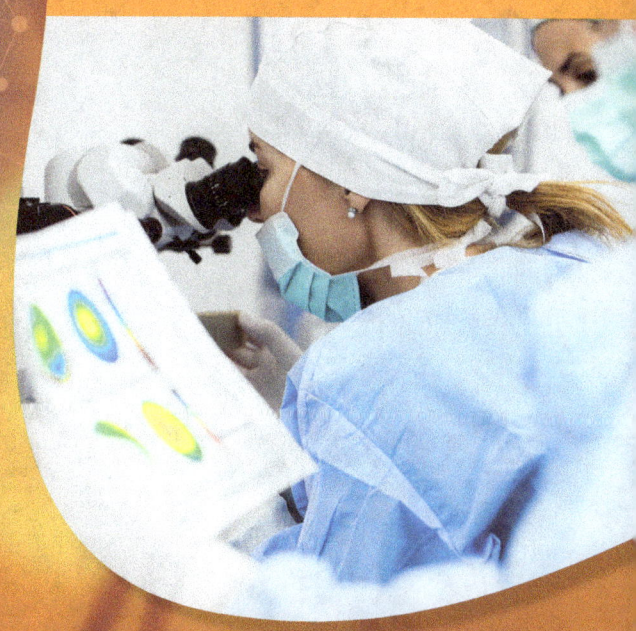

Retinal implants do not restore full vision, because they cannot replicate the function of retinal cells that help identify images. After surgery, the patient must learn to interpret the new signals as shapes and objects. This takes time. It cannot create a detailed picture, but it may help a blind person find their way around obstacles or even read a large print book.

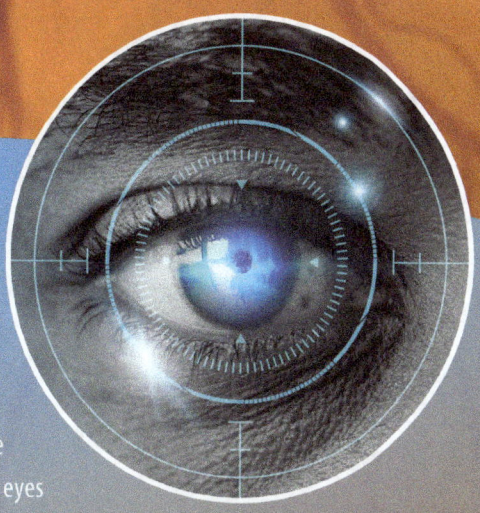

A different vision

Right now, retinal implants only work for people who lose sight due to retinal damage. People who were born blind or have injuries to the eye or optic nerve are not helped by retinal implants. Scientists are researching other kinds of implants and even artificial eyes that can restore vision to anyone with vision loss.

Reusable ROCKETS:
Making spaceflight less wasteful

Imagine if an airline threw away the aircraft after every flight. That would be wasteful and expensive. Yet until recently, this has been how spaceflight operated. Single-use rockets fly just once, then fall into the ocean or burn up in the atmosphere. Today, engineers are building rockets that can fly up to space and then return to Earth to be reused.

How do reusable rockets work? To escape Earth's gravity and reach outer space, rockets require a lot of thrust. Most use a series of small rockets, or "stages," stacked on top of one another. In conventional rockets, the first stages are discarded after their fuel has run out.

Reusable rockets usually have two stages. The first stage sends the rocket to the edge of space. Here, the second stage separates and fires its engine to take it into space. But instead of falling into the sea, the first stage flips around, flies back to Earth, and lands on a platform.

One of the most famous reusable rockets is Falcon 9, built by the aerospace company SpaceX. It has nine engines to control its descent and land upright. The rocket's fins help steer the rocket to the landing pad—a floating barge out at sea. Four legs deploy to absorb the force of landing. An onboard computer controls the engines, fins, and legs. Sensors feed the computer information on the craft's velocity, orientation, and altitude, as well as changes in air pressure and wind speed.

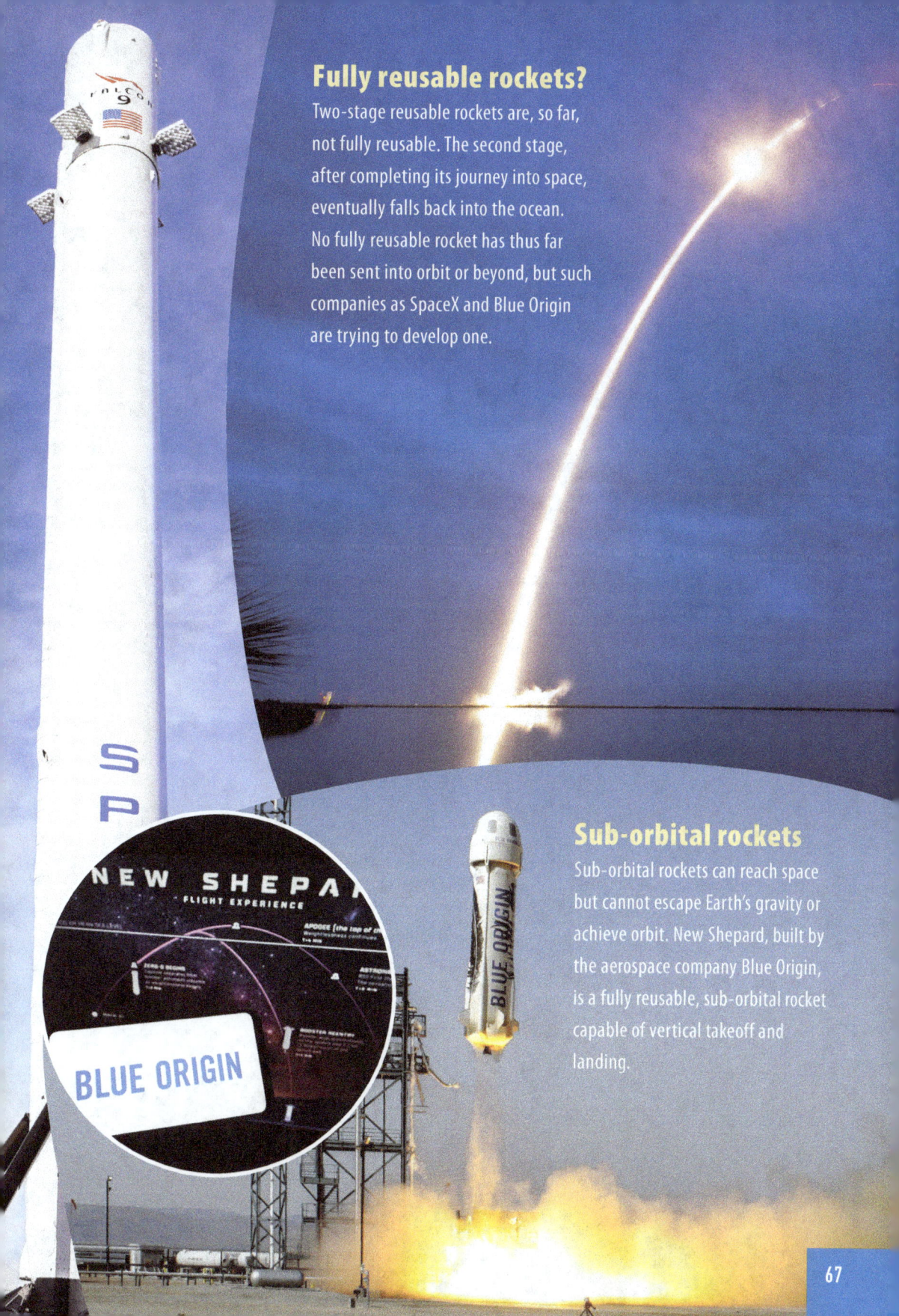

Fully reusable rockets?

Two-stage reusable rockets are, so far, not fully reusable. The second stage, after completing its journey into space, eventually falls back into the ocean. No fully reusable rocket has thus far been sent into orbit or beyond, but such companies as SpaceX and Blue Origin are trying to develop one.

Sub-orbital rockets

Sub-orbital rockets can reach space but cannot escape Earth's gravity or achieve orbit. New Shepard, built by the aerospace company Blue Origin, is a fully reusable, sub-orbital rocket capable of vertical takeoff and landing.

Satellite INTERNET:
Connected to the sky

You may use the internet every day, but have you ever thought about how it reaches you? Most internet travels through a network of fiber-optic cables, even if you connect to it over Wi-Fi. But a network of satellites may soon change that.

Satellite internet uses orbiting satellites to send and receive data signals. This allows the internet to reach remote areas that don't have internet cables.

Internet satellites sit in a geostationary orbit about 22,240 miles (35,790 kilometers) above Earth. Each satellite remains over one point on Earth, and the whole network can reach every part of Earth's surface. This makes it useful for ships, aircraft, remote research stations, and oil rigs. Satellite internet could also help emergency responders stay connected when wired internet is disrupted, such as during natural disasters.

Satellite internet does have a slight signal delay, or latency, because even traveling at light speed, the signals have a long way to go between a satellite and the ground. This could be a problem for online gaming or video conferencing. However, as technology improves this may become less of a problem.

Satellite internet also requires a satellite dish to send and receive data. These must be kept clean and pointed in the right direction. Some companies design their dishes to withstand rain, dust, snow, and temperatures as cold as -220 °F (-300 °C). Some even come with heaters to melt snow on the dish.

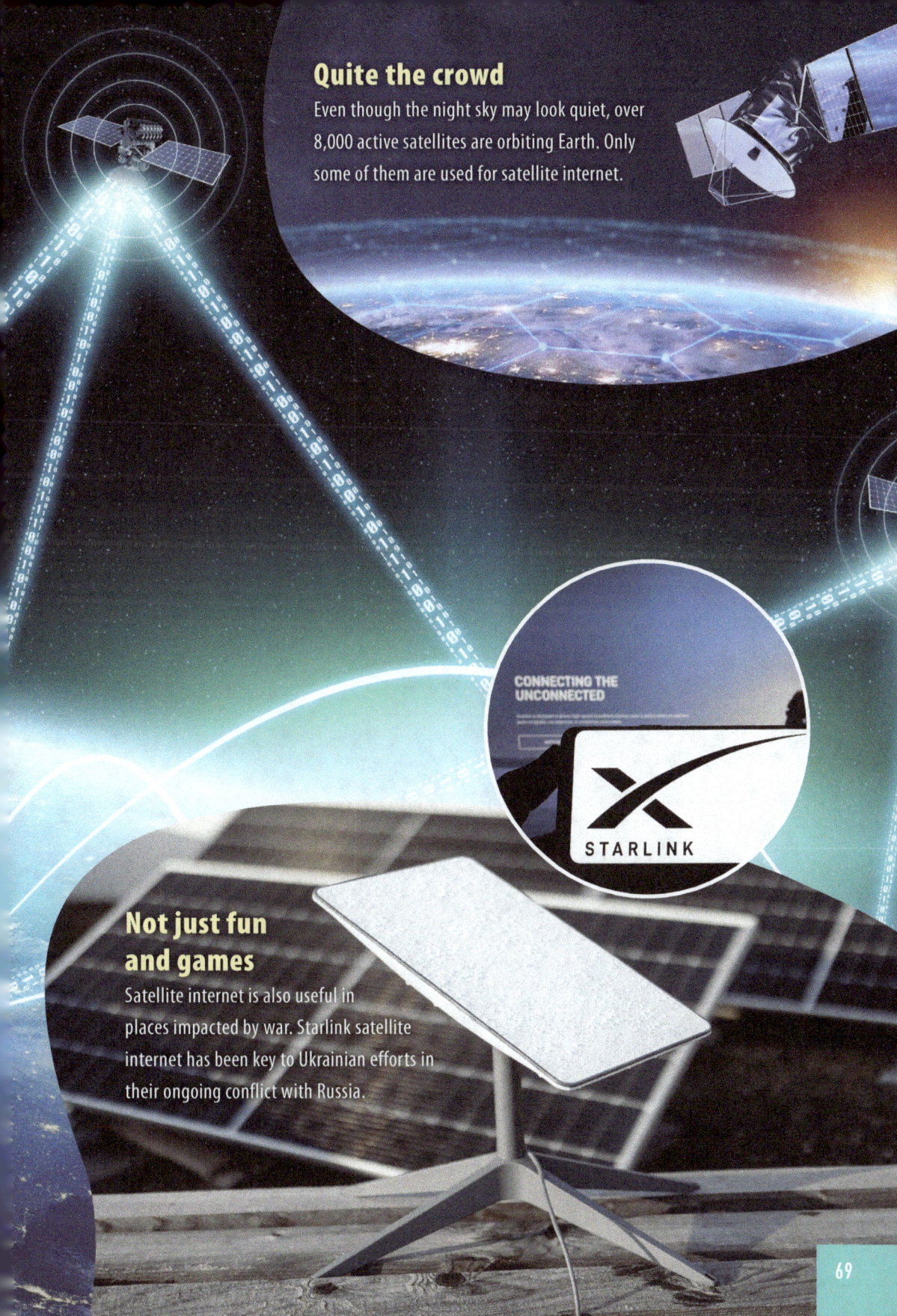

Quite the crowd
Even though the night sky may look quiet, over 8,000 active satellites are orbiting Earth. Only some of them are used for satellite internet.

Not just fun and games
Satellite internet is also useful in places impacted by war. Starlink satellite internet has been key to Ukrainian efforts in their ongoing conflict with Russia.

SOLID-STATE LIDAR:
Helping robots navigate

A self-driving car applies its brakes when the car in front slows down. A drone rises to avoid hitting an electricity pylon. A hospital robot turns a corner on its way to deliver medicine to a patient. All these machines navigate their environment using a technology called lidar.

Lidar stands for *l*ight *d*etection *a*nd *r*anging. A lidar device emits pulses of laser light. The light strikes the surface of a nearby object and bounces back to a sensor. The sensor calculates its distance from the object based on how long it took the light to return. A computer on board uses these measurements to generate a detailed, three-dimensional view of its surroundings.

Traditional lidar devices are mechanical. They have a rotating platform so the light pulses can be sent out in all directions. This means they can be confused if the platform shakes. A new kind of solid-state lidar has no moving parts, making the devices smaller, less expensive, and more reliable.

Solid-state lidar uses electronics to control and direct the laser pulses. It cannot capture the full 360 degrees of its surroundings, but the latest versions have a field of view of up to 270 degrees. Solid state lidar devices also have faster processing speeds, allowing a vehicle's computer to make quick decisions as it travels.

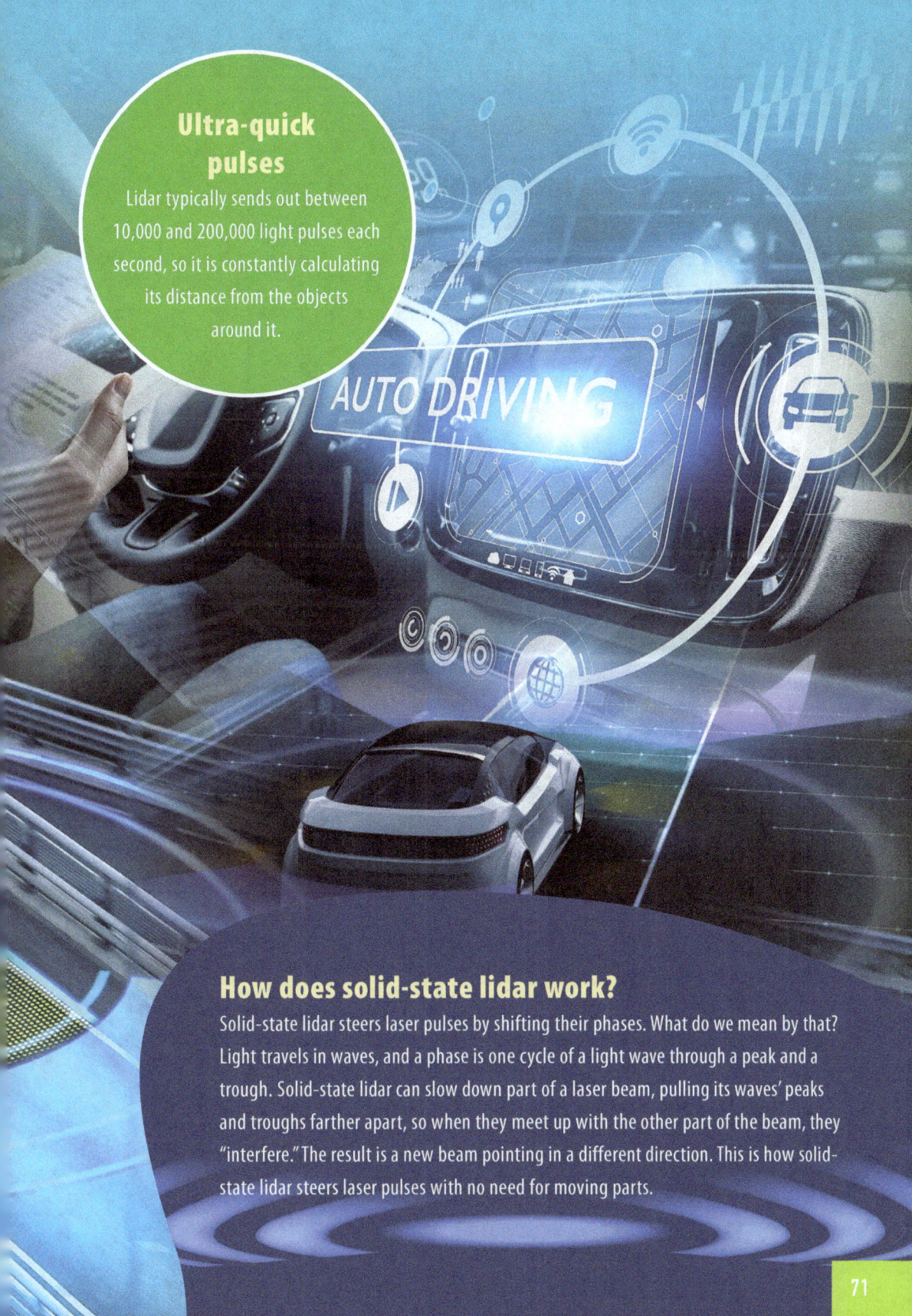

Ultra-quick pulses
Lidar typically sends out between 10,000 and 200,000 light pulses each second, so it is constantly calculating its distance from the objects around it.

How does solid-state lidar work?
Solid-state lidar steers laser pulses by shifting their phases. What do we mean by that? Light travels in waves, and a phase is one cycle of a light wave through a peak and a trough. Solid-state lidar can slow down part of a laser beam, pulling its waves' peaks and troughs farther apart, so when they meet up with the other part of the beam, they "interfere." The result is a new beam pointing in a different direction. This is how solid-state lidar steers laser pulses with no need for moving parts.

SPACE CROPS:
Food for the future

Could astronauts grow their own food in space? Many space missions have taken plants and seeds into orbit around Earth to try to find out.

Cultivating crops in space helps researchers understand the effects of microgravity and radiation on plant growth. In 2022, scientists on China's Tiangong Space Station (TSS) tested out space farming with rice and thale cress plants.

The seeds were cultivated in a sealed artificial environment, like a greenhouse. But the plants experienced weightlessness and the increased radiation of space. Over 120 days, the seeds successfully sprouted, grew, flowered, and produced seeds in space. In December 2022, the plants were harvested and the seeds returned to Earth. Scientists observed only a few slight differences between the rice and thale cress plants grown in space compared to those grown on Earth.

Scientists on the International Space Station (ISS) and TSS have conducted experiments with dozens of different plants. In 2020, China sent rice seeds to the moon and back. Other experiments have helped develop new varieties of broccoli, peppers, and flowers. Back on Earth, scientists have managed to *germinate* (sprout) plants in soil made from moon dust. This experiment shows that it may be possible to grow crops beyond Earth—perhaps on Mars!

Scientists hope that growing plants in space will provide a steady supply of fresh food for humans on long space missions. Space crops could also generate breathable oxygen and remove carbon dioxide from a spacecraft.

Generating mutations

Over 30 years, China has sent rice and other plant seeds on brief space trips, where they are exposed to the higher radiation of low Earth orbit. Scientists then look for mutations that could increase crop yields or disease resistance. In these missions, the seeds were flown to space but grown back on Earth.

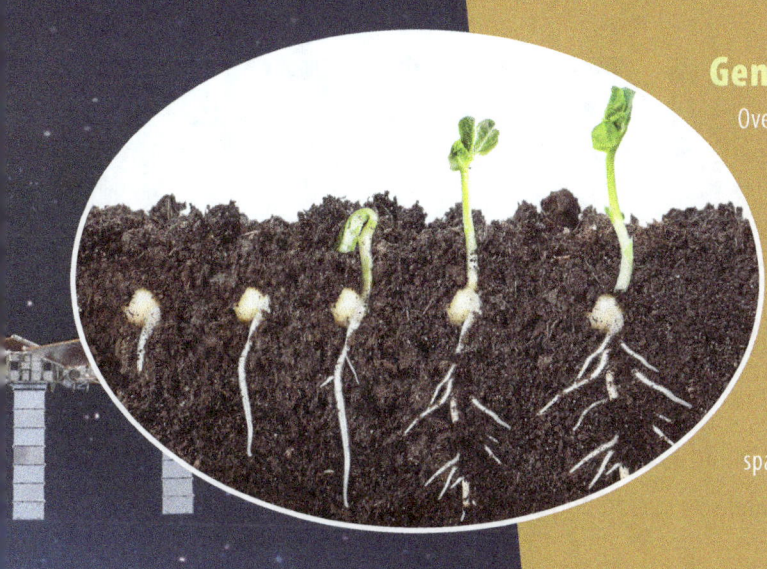

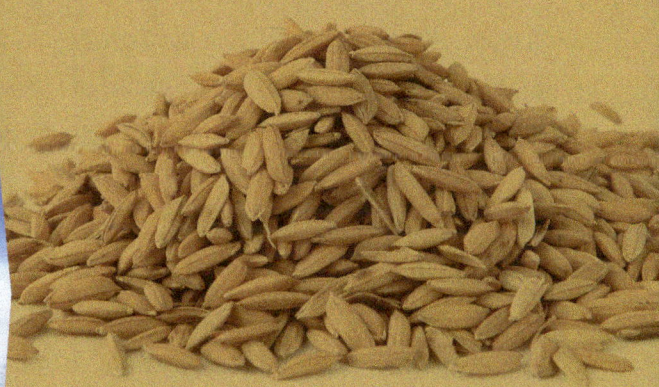

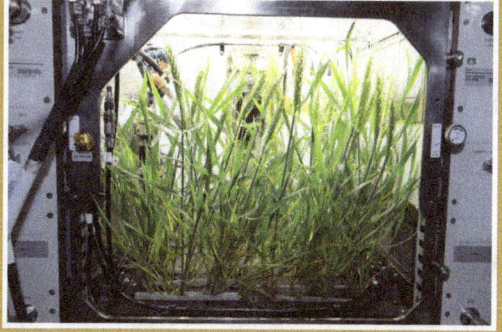

Space peppers

Several countries have developed new varieties of crops based on genetic mutations that were generated in space. The first space-bred crop was a sweet pepper! It was bigger and more disease-resistant than peppers bred on Earth.

TELEHEALTH:
No more waiting rooms with virtual healthcare

Are you sneezing, coughing, or running a fever? The last thing you want to do is head out to see the doctor and risk spreading your cold.

With telehealth, you can visit your doctor over your computer or smartphone. Telehealth is healthcare provided remotely. It can include video conferencing, phone calls, and email with healthcare professionals.

The first people to have their health monitored remotely were astronauts in the 1960's. The United States National Aeronautics and Space Administration (NASA) used sensors to monitor astronauts' blood pressure, heart rate, and temperature. Astronauts could talk to a doctor over radio link if a medical problem arose.

In 2002, a NASA surgeon co-founded Teladoc, the first national telehealth provider. Telehealth became popular during the COVID-19 pandemic, when hospitals were full and people wanted to stay home to stop the spread of the virus.

Many medical services, including mental health therapy, physical therapy, and patient wellness checks, can be done remotely. Fitness trackers and other devices help remote care providers monitor patients. People with diabetes might log their glucose levels for their doctor to see. Others might wear heart rate monitors for a cardiologist.

Sinusitis assistance

A 2014 study showed sinusitis was the most common diagnosis made through telehealth. Sinusitis is an infection or inflammation of the nasal cavity. Around 20 percent of all diagnoses were for sinusitis!

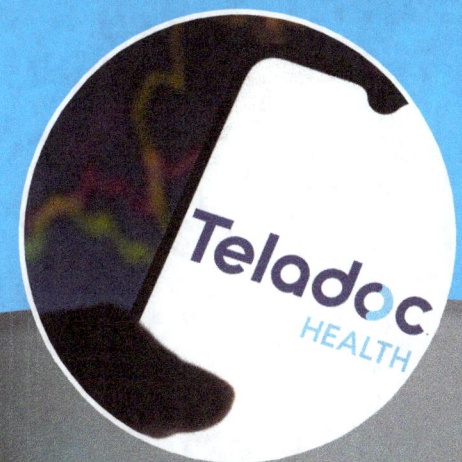

Telehealth allows patients to communicate with a physician without having to wait for an office appointment or travel long distances. Doctors can also get second opinions quickly by sending information to colleagues.

With most telehealth systems, patients can log in to a secure site to video conference, message, and schedule appointments with their healthcare team. Telehealth keeps expanding!

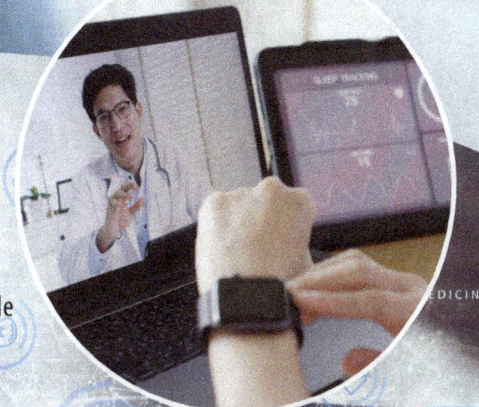

Too far for a house call

Today, only about 1 in 10 American physicians work outside of cities. That means there is a shortage of doctors in rural communities. Telehealth can help people in these places find the care they need remotely.

Wireless capsule endoscopy:

Exploring the body with a pill

When something goes wrong inside the body, doctors want to take a look to see what's causing the problem. Now, tiny cameras in a pill are allowing them see inside without surgery, using a tool called *wireless capsule endoscopy*.

Endoscopy means *looking inside the body*. The capsule holds a tiny camera. The patient swallows the capsule, and it goes through the digestive tract. On its way, it snaps more pictures than an enthusiastic tourist. It transmits these images wirelessly to a recording device.

Old-fashioned endoscopy involves inserting a tube called an *endoscope* into a patient's mouth or another opening. The tube has a camera at one end, allowing doctors to examine the colon, stomach, and upper small bowel. Unfortunately, the endoscope is uncomfortable and can only go so far.

Capsule endoscopy can get to such hard-to-reach places as the small intestine. It can help doctors locate the source of bleeding, inflammation, or tumors.

Gut friendly

There are not many nonfood objects that a doctor would advise you to swallow. A medical capsule is one exception. Some capsules can monitor breathing, heart rate, and temperature. Capsules can also deliver precision drug doses to treat gastrointestinal (GI) disorders.

Capsule endoscopy can also show how the digestive tract reacts to *gluten*, a substance in wheat flour. This helps doctors to diagnose celiac disease.

Capsules that could take video were introduced in 2001. The camera is just millimeters wide—a fraction of an inch. Natural muscle contractions move the camera along on its all-night tour of the intestines. The camera leaves the body on its own in about 24 hours.

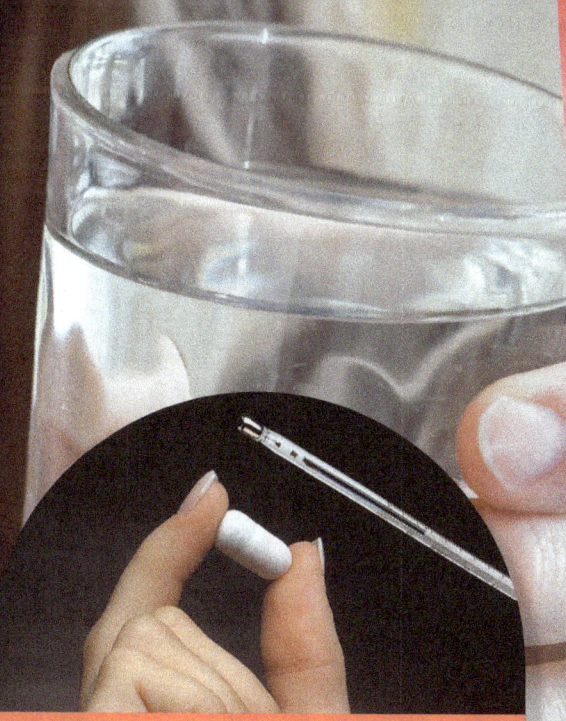

Temperature extremes
This "thermometer pill" was invented by researchers at Johns Hopkins University and NASA to monitor the body temperatures of astronauts. Athletes and firefighters also use them to watch for signs of dangerous heat exhaustion.

Index

adenine (molecule), 36
aerogels, 6-7
antibodies, 54
Argus II (medical device), 15, 64
artificial intelligence (AI), 8-11

bacteria, 5, 7, 22, 47
Berger, Hans, 17
bionics, 14-15, 61
black holes, 28-29, 51
Blue Origin (company), 67
body temperature, 41, 77
brain-computer interface (BCI), 16-17

Cas9 (molecule), 22-23, 25
CERN (European Organization for Nuclear Research), 48
Charpentier, Emmanuelle, 23
ChatGPT, 9
chromosomes, 35
cloning, 18-19
cloud computing, 20-21
cochlear implants, 14
continuous glucose monitor (CGM), 56
COVID-19, 40, 54, 74

Cpf1 (molecule), 25
CRISPR, 22-25
crops, 22, 24, 72-73
CubeSats, 26-27
cytosine (molecule), 36

dark matter, 48
decoherence, 63
Deep Blue (computer), 9
diabetes, 38, 56, 74
DNA (molecule), 18, 22-25, 34-38, 55
Dolly (cloned sheep), 18
Doudna, Jennifer, 23

Einstein, Albert, 28, 51
endoscopy, 76-77
enzymes, 22, 25, 37
Event Horizon Telescope (EHT), 28-29
exoskeletons, 15

Falcon 9 (rocket), 66
Food and Drug Administration (FDA), 30-31

General Magic (company), 21
generative adversarial network (GAN), 11

genes, 18-19, 22-25, 30-31, 34-39
genetically modified organisms (GMO's), 30-31
Genographic Project, 35
glucose, 56, 74
González, Gabriela, 51
gravitational waves, 50-51
gravity, 28, 48, 50-51, 66-67
guanine (molecule), 36

Higgs, Peter, 49
Higgs boson, 49
Hoffman, David, 21
holograms, 32-33
Human Genome Project (HGP), 38-39

infrared waves, 40-45
insulin, 56-57
International Space Station (ISS), 72
internet, 20, 68-69

James Webb Space Telescope (JWST), 42-45
Johns Hopkins University, 77

Karikó, Katalin, 55
Kasparov, Garry, 9

lab-grown meat, 46-47
Large Hadron Collider (LHC), 48-49
Laser Interferometer Gravitational-Wave Observatory (LIGO), 50-51
lasers, 32, 40, 50-51, 70-71
lidar, 70-71
liver, 12-13

machine learning, 8, 60
Mars Cube One (space mission), 27
mass (property of matter), 49
Matsumura, Kenneth, 12
McCarthy, John, 9
Messier 87 (galaxy), 29
metamaterials, 52-53
metasurfaces, 53
microarray chip, 36
monkeys (cloned), 18-19
motion parallax, 32
myoelectric prostheses, 58-60

National Aeronautics and Space Administration (NASA), 7, 42, 45, 74, 77
Neuralink (company), 17
NextMind (company), 16

Omnipod (medical device), 56-57
Orion Visual Cortical Prosthesis System, 15

Pairwise (company), 24
Pepper, John Henry, 33
polymerase chain reaction, 37
proprioception, 61
prosthetics, 14-16
proteins, 22, 54

quantum computing, 62-63
qubits, 62-63

radio waves, 53
retinal implants, 64-65
RNA (molecule), 22, 54-55
rockets, 43, 66-67

Sagittarius A* (black hole), 29
satellites, 26-27, 68-69
sinusitis, 75

sound, 14, 53
SpaceX (company), 66-67
Standard Model, 48-49
Starlink (group of satellites), 69
sun shields, 42
superposition, 62-63

Teladoc (company), 74
telehealth, 74-75
thermometers, 40-41
three-dimensional (3D) printing, 4-5, 59
thymine (molecule), 36
Tiangong Space Station (TSS), 72
Turing, Alan, 9

Ukraine War, 69
Utah Bionic Leg, 61

vaccines, 54-55
very-long baseline interferometry, 28
video processing unit (VPU), 64
viruses, 5, 22, 74

Webb, James, 45

Acknowledgments

Cover	© PopTika/Shutterstock; © Cryptographer/Shutterstock; © Gorodenkoff/Shutterstock; © muratart/Shutterstock; © Artemis Diana, Shutterstock; © natrot/Shutterstock; © NicoElNino/Shutterstock; © NewJadsada/Shutterstock; © Jim Barber, Shutterstock; © khoamartin/Shutterstock
4-5	© guteksk7/Shutterstock; © Sergey Kolesnikov, Shutterstock; © luchschenF/Shutterstock
6-7	© LuYago/Shutterstock; © Alones/Shutterstock; © LuYago/Shutterstock; © Zay Nyi Nyi, Shutterstock; © Jurik Peter, Shutterstock
8-9	© NicoElNino/Shutterstock; © FAMILY STOCK/Shutterstock
10-11	© plotplot/Shutterstock; © Ryzhi/Shutterstock; © archy13/Shutterstock
12-13	© MattL_Images/Shutterstock; © Explode/Shutterstock; © Marko Aliaksandr, Shutterstock; © Ben Schonewille, Shutterstock
14-15	© Second Sight; © PHOTOCREO Michal Bednarek/Shutterstock; © Unai Huizi Photography/Shutterstock; © Elnur/Shutterstock; © Ivan Shenets, Shutterstock; © Tum ZzzzZ/Shutterstock
16-17	© Volodymyr Burdiak, Shutterstock; © Gorodenkoff/Shutterstock; © Followtheflow/Shutterstock; © KwangSoo Kim/Shutterstock; © Red Confidential/Shutterstock; © yurakrasil/Shutterstock
18-19	© Sun Qiang and Poo Muming, Chinese Academy of Sciences/AP Photo; © Steph Couvrette, Shutterstock; © SquareMotion/Shutterstock
20-21	© Connect world/Shutterstock; © jijomathaidesigners/Shutterstock; © one photo/Shutterstock; © vs148/Shutterstock
22-23	© Butusova Elena, Shutterstock; © Gohang/Shutterstock; © Yurchanka Siarhei, Shutterstock
24-25	© AtlasStudio/Shutterstock; © PopTika/Shutterstock; © Immersion Imagery/Shutterstock; © Alexander Raths, Shutterstock
26-27	© Phillip van Zyl/Shutterstock; © BLACKDAY/Shutterstock
28-29	© Boris Rabtsevich, Shutterstock; © mapush/Shutterstock; © Vadim Sadovski, Shutterstock; © Triff/Shutterstock; © joingate/Shutterstock
30-31	© ArtemisDiana/Shutterstock; © CeltStudio/Shutterstock; © PeopleImages.com - Yuri A/Shutterstock; © Jesus Cervantes, Shutterstock; © Polawat Klinkulabhirun, Shutterstock
32-33	© Paul Prescott, Shutterstock; © Migren art/Shutterstock; © Peshkova/Shutterstock; © khoamartin/Shutterstock; © Gorodenkoff/Shutterstock
34-35	© Billion Photos/Shutterstock; © natrot/Shutterstock; © Mind Pixell/Shutterstock
36-37	© luchschenF/Shutterstock; © Dmitry Kovalchuk, Shutterstock; © Microgen/Shutterstock; © Frogella/Shutterstock
38-39	© angellodeco/Shutterstock; © WinWin artlab/Shutterstock; © gopixa/Shutterstock; © Billion Photos/Shutterstock
40-41	© pixinoo/Shutterstock; © VladyslaV Travel photo/Shutterstock; © thecloudysunny/Shutterstock; © Peakstock/Shutterstock
42-43	© muratart/Shutterstock; © lotos_land/Shutterstock
44-45	© Dima Zel, Shutterstock; © BEST-BACKGROUNDS/Shutterstock; © Artsiom P/Shutterstock
46-47	© Zapp2Photo/Shutterstock; © TopMicrobialStock/Shutterstock
48-49	© sakkmesterke/Shutterstock; © D-VISIONS/Shutterstock; © Kapustin Igor, Shutterstock; © Dominionart/Shutterstock
50-51	© vchal/Shutterstock; © sakkmesterke/Shutterstock; © Roberto Michel, Shutterstock; © canbedone/Shutterstock
52-53	© luchschenF/Shutterstock; © frantic00/Shutterstock; © Jim Barber, Shutterstock; © Dmitry Steshenko, Shutterstock; © leungchopan/Shutterstock
54-55	© gyn9037/Shutterstock; © Dmitry Kalinovsky, Shutterstock; © Cryptographer/Shutterstock; © Michael Oddi, Shutterstock
56-57	© Maria Wan, Shutterstock; © Irina Shatilova, Shutterstock
58-59	© NewJadsada/Shutterstock; © Hodoimg/Shutterstock; © 1st footage/Shutterstock; © luchschenF/Shutterstock
60-61	© Pressmaster/Shutterstock; © Gorodenkoff/Shutterstock; © Dean Drobot, Shutterstock; © SeventyFour/Shutterstock
62-63	© Audio und werbung/Shutterstock; © metamorworks/Shutterstock; © Bartlomiej K. Wroblewski, Shutterstock; © Funtap/Shutterstock
64-65	© VesnaArt/Shutterstock; © DuxX/Shutterstock; © Kateryna Kon/Shutterstock; © Rawpixel.com/Shutterstock; © Elnur/Shutterstock
66-67	© T. Schneider/Shutterstock; © Aqeela_Image/Shutterstock; © YMZK-Photo/Shutterstock; © Blue Origin; © Sundry Photography/Shutterstock
68-69	© sdecoret/Shutterstock; © Ross Helen, Shutterstock; © Wirestock Creators/Shutterstock; © NicoElNino/Shutterstock
70-71	© Gorodenkoff/Shutterstock; © metamorworks/Shutterstock; © O-IAHI/Shutterstock
72-73	© sevenke/Shutterstock; NASA; © Dima Zel, Shutterstock; © alexdov/Shutterstock
74-75	© TippaPatt/Shutterstock; © rafapress/Shutterstock; © PeopleImages.com - Yuri A/Shutterstock; © Chay_Tee/Shutterstock
76-77	© shutterIk/Shutterstock; © Kzenon/Shutterstock; © Magic mine/Shutterstock
78-81	© Shutterstock

www.ingramcontent.com/pod-product-compliance
Lightning Source LLC
Chambersburg PA
CBHW080923180426
43192CB00040B/2666